*f*P

FREE PRESS
A Division of Simon & Schuster, Inc.
1230 Avenue of the Americas
New York, NY 10020

FREE PRESS and colophon are trademarks
of Simon & Schuster, Inc.

Designed by Julie Schroeder

Manufactured in the United States of America

1   3   5   7   9   10   8   6   4   2

Library of Congress Cataloging-in-Publication
Data Control Number: 2005040625

ISBN 0-7432-7081-9

For information regarding special discounts for bulk purchases,
please contact Simon & Schuster Special Sales
at 1-800-456-6798 or business@simonandschuster.com

easure

E YOURSELF
MA
ATE
BE

aya Rodale

RESS

TORONTO • SYDNEY

This book is dedicated to Mary and Eve

Pleasure:

A feeling of satisfaction or joy, a person's will or desire.

CONTENTS

INTRODUCTION

THIS IS A BOOK ABOUT THE POWER OF STORIES TO CHANGE YOUR LIFE

It's about stories we know deep in our soul, but have forgotten. It's about discovering the reasons why we forgot them, and remembering them again—and seeing them in a new way. It's about why our culture looks down on those happily ending romances and fairy tales that little girls love and women secretly crave. This book is about why we let our children watch violence on TV, yet sex is strictly forbidden. It's about our story as women—mothers, daughters, friends, journeying together on a long, adventure-filled, and sometimes frightening path. It's the story of many women who you may or may not have heard of, but who have paved the way for all of us in revolutionary ways—in spite of tremendous odds.

These stories have already changed our lives and continue to, so we want to share our own story with you to show you some possible paths to take. But the true magic happens when you create your own story, which this book will help you do.

What's the main story that we've forgotten? It's the story of pleasure. How we lost it. Where we can find it again. It's the story of why pleasure often makes us feel guilty, as if we don't deserve it. It's about why we truly *do* deserve it, why it matters, and why it's so easy for us as women to say, every day, as we are helping others, "It's my pleasure," but so hard for us to say to ourselves "It's MY pleasure." This story is about a revolution in your attitude about yourself and about pleasure. It's about taking action to create positive change in your life and in the world. And, it's about appreciating the tremendous, wonderful change that has already occurred. Finally, it's about believing that maybe we can create a happy ending after all.

HOW I TRIPPED AND STUMBLED ONTO
THE PATH OF PLEASURE—MARIA

When I was thirty-five I quit my job.

You have to understand how scandalous this was. I had been designated the heir of my family's publishing business by my father, who had died seven years earlier. Until my mother decided to retire, which she vehemently vowed never to do, she was in charge of the company; then it would be my "turn." I was expected to work my way up the ladder, rung by rung, proving myself to the Guys (and to the occasional Girl-Guy, which is a woman who wants to be one of the Guys) along the way (none of whom, I realized later, really wanted me to succeed). I'd been climbing persistently since I was thirteen when my parents forced me to work at the company to keep me out of trouble after school (the joke was on them).

When I was thirty-five I developed a fibroid the size of a golf ball. I thought this was ironic since, as a woman in business, it always had irked me that men went off on any sunny day to play golf and called it work. I read a book called *Women's Bodies, Women's Wisdom* by Christiane Northrup, which said that fibroids were the physical manifestation of unborn creativity stuck inside us. She hit a nerve.

My job title at the time was creative director, but there was absolutely nothing creative about it. Most of my time was spent on budgets and personality conflicts. I managed a department of seventy people who were accountable to persnickety, often small-minded "clients" who always wanted completely safe but "out-of-the-box" thinking. Of course, there's no such thing. Plus, I oversaw our direct marketing business. There is something depressing about creating a mailing piece that 97 percent of people who receive it throw in the trash (if you are successful).

At one of our management retreats, a guest speaker urged us to write our own obituaries in order to get in touch with our true desires. That night in bed, while the Guys were at the bar getting drunk, I wrote mine. It became totally clear to me that I was on the wrong path in life.

I wanted to be a writer. When I died, I wanted to have "author of . . ." behind my name. But all I had written to date were memos, direct mail copy, and dozens of journal entries filled with bad poetry.

So I quit. I had been married a few years before and was thinking about having more kids. I also was the parent of a fifteen-year-old girl who I had had "out of wedlock" when I was twenty. (More on that later.) By the time I made my decision to leave my job and set my last day of work, I actually was two and one-half months pregnant.

I will never forget the horrible moment right before I was to speak to a room full of seventy people waiting to hear my farewell speech. I had run to the bathroom, saw blood, and knew I was miscarrying the baby. With toilet paper stuck between my legs, I went back into the room and gave my speech.

The first month of my "leave of absence," as my mother called it, was spent recovering from a D&C to remove the dead fetus. I bled for the whole month.

Then I tried to get in touch with my inner fibroid to figure out what it wanted to be. I decided to write a book on organic gardening, something I am very passionate about.

My grandfather, J. I. Rodale, invented organic gardening in 1942. His ideas were an integral part of my upbringing. As part of my research I decided to read what he and my father, Robert Rodale, had written. My grandfather's books were eccentric, funny, crazy, and brilliant. He got into trouble for the stuff he said, but I was shocked at how much of it was finally proven to be true. Among his insights: smoking causes cancer (he was the first one to publicly claim this at a time when doctors were featured in cigarette ads); and exercise and nutrition prevent disease (again, he was one of the first to make the claim back in the 1940s).

My father's writing was different. His books were filled with dire predictions . . . like if we don't ride bicycles instead of cars there will be no oil left in twenty years, and we will all be doomed. Given that I was reading his book thirty years after he wrote that, and cars were bigger and more prevalent than ever, I felt kind of embarrassed for him. But his passion for change led him to do many great things for the world— including launching the first long-term studies into organic versus modern agriculture—so I didn't hold it against him.

It was while reading one of my father's books that I realized that most of the organic and environmental movement was using a fear-based, doomsday method to motivate people to change. If we didn't do what they said, we would all starve and strangle ourselves in our own filth. That's if we didn't blow ourselves to smithereens first. There was even a prejudice against beauty. If it was beautiful, they must have used chemicals, or it must be evil, the thinking of the time went. Ugliness and frugality were the ultimate virtues, and "simplicity" was the code word.

But real positive change seemed to be happening in the organic movement in food. Gourmet food. Alice Waters and her restaurant Chez Panisse, in Berkeley, California, started it in the 1970s. She made organic food taste so good that the appreciative "foodies" made it cool. Next thing you knew, all the high-end chefs were going organic, and Whole Foods markets became one of the hottest growth stocks around.

The first time I walked into a Whole Foods I cried. Finally, someone had gotten it right. I tried to imagine what my grandfather would have thought—back then if you wanted organic food you had to grow it yourself and endure the ridicule of your neighbors. Sixty years later you could enter a paradise of pleasure and buy almost anything organic you wanted.

That was the first time I tripped and stumbled onto the path of pleasure. But I still didn't recognize it fully, nor did I accept that it was my true path. But I was beginning to see one of the first truths about pleasure, which is that pleasure is a better motivator for change than fear.

Fast-forward five years. I've written a gardening book and a laundry book. I've had a healthy baby girl (and two more miscarriages). I've realized I am an alcoholic and given up drinking. I've returned to the family business and led a massive management change along with my mother, which resulted in most of the Guys leaving for good. (This change was just in time, too, since our business was in deep trouble and the banks were breathing down our necks.) I've launched a magazine called *Organic Style*, the aim of which is to seduce people into doing the right thing rather than scaring them. The only downside then was that it was costing more money than we had.

Was it pleasurable? Hell no! I actually had people walk up to me in the local supermarket and say they would never want to be me. Frankly, I didn't want to be me, either.

Here is what kept me alive during that time . . . romance novels. At the end of an excruciating day I couldn't come home and drown my sorrows in a martini or bottle of red wine anymore. But I could escape to a place where the women were strong and the men were good-looking. Something about their stories of victory over adversity, people following their true hearts instead of society's rules, and the transformational power of love gave me the strength to wake up another day and keep at it.

And yet . . . I was embarrassed for myself. No one else I knew read romances, or at least admitted to it. In the publishing world, of which I was a member, they were considered trash, drivel that was beneath the nose of anyone who had any intelligence or sophistication. If I had had any taste I would have been perfectly happy reading stories of rape, murder, incest, the meaninglessness and inhumanity of life . . . much of which is called literary fiction. Occasionally, a Jane Austen book was allowed into this lofty circle, but only if it was read as social satire rather than romance.

The more research I did into the genre and history of romance the angrier I got. Here was the largest selling genre of fiction, and it was completely disregarded by those "in the know" as not being worth the paper it was printed on—except to all the people making so much money off it and all the women, like me, who found hope and inspiration in it.

Out of curiosity, I attended a Romance Writers of America conference. I needed to see for myself who was behind all this stuff. Were they the miserable outcasts of society? Were the writers ugly, bitter spinsters who never got any for themselves and so had to invent it on the page? Were the readers, as one literary agent had described them, white trash women with cigarette butts hanging out of their mouths laboring over the ironing board?

As I entered the lobby of the New York City Hilton I felt as though I had entered an alternative reality. First of all, I had never heard such a high-pitched buzz of excitement inside a hotel lobby. The chirping was deafening. There were old women, young women, stunningly gorgeous women and not so pretty women, thin women in mini skirts, fat women in long flowing tartan plaids. There were overtly sexy women and a few who looked like those librarians before they let down their hair and took off their glasses and were totally hot. But they shared one common factor—they all seemed excited, smart, and

FREE. They had made their choice to do what they loved, and they were reveling in it.

That was the second time I tripped and stumbled onto the path of pleasure. But I still wasn't quite sure it was right for me . . . although I was definitely starting to feel more joy and less guilt about reading romances. In fact, I imagined myself as a heroine of my own story. I had learned another important clue to pleasure: Optimism and hope feel good. Cynicism and despair feel bad. I chose to feel good.

The third and final trip and fall was a long, slow, jagged tumble that had been going on my whole life, a sort of fall from grace, search-for-God-in-everything, spiritual journey. My father was a lapsed Jew. My mother was a lapsed Lutheran. I had the sneaking suspicion that there must be some commonality that would unite all the religions, but I was kind of frustrated and angry that they all seem to have been built by men, for men, with their highest ideal, in the case of Christianity, being a celibate man (talk about lack of romance!).

In an Asian religion class I took the year after I had given birth to my daughter, Maya, the teacher spoke of the highest ideal of Buddhism and Hinduism being renunciation. She undoubtedly oversimplified the philosophies, yet I could barely contain my horror. What an irresponsible, selfish way to worship God, I thought. Yet part of why I had decided to have Maya rather than abort my unplanned teenage pregnancy was my belief in karma and the sacredness of all life.

Later, I started reading about religious history and was absolutely appalled by the corruption, competition, genocide, power struggles, countless episodes of heads being chopped off and burnings at the stake. And New Age religions seemed populated by creepy people who were more concerned with elevating themselves to guru-hood. No religion seemed to have a clean, honest past that I felt I could commit to. None. I wanted no part of any of them.

And yet, I felt very spiritual and connected to the universe. I never stopped believing in some sort of higher being. But I needed an anchor. A role model. A pioneer to lead me onto the path of pleasure for good. I found her one day while I was cleaning. Seriously.

Here is what happened. My husband is happily and devotedly Roman Catholic. I had agreed to marry him in a Catholic ceremony but also had his agreement that I didn't have to convert. I found it funny that the church had no problem with me being an unwed mother—but if I had been married and divorced with children, I would have had to get an annulment in order to marry him. I guess since the Virgin Mary was an unwed mother, it made it okay. Anyway, I was down on the floor cleaning when I found the following prayer on a magnet stuck to the radiator. It was the prayer that the high school football team my husband had played on twenty years earlier would say before every game. At the time Maya was about nine and entering a more independent phase of her childhood. I was full of fear. I worried obsessively any time she wasn't with me and was terrified that something terrible would happen to her. I read the prayer:

MEMORARE

Remember, O most compassionate Virgin Mary, that never was it known that anyone who fled to your protection, implored your assistance, or sought your intercession, was left unaided. Inspired with this confidence, we fly unto you, O Virgin of Virgins, Our Mother; to you we come; before you we kneel sinful and sorrowful. O Mother of the Word Incarnate, despise not our petitions, but in your clemency hear and answer them. Amen.

Because I actually was kneeling as I read it (since it was stuck to the radiator for God knows what reason!), I had a moment of enlightenment—a religious epiphany. It was sort of a "DUH!—If you want something, ask Mom, don't ask Dad!"

Then I started finding Marys everywhere and bringing them home. I'd buy old, cracked Virgin Marys at flea markets for a dollar. Some were even as cheap as ten cents. I felt like I was rescuing her from abandonment and degradation. I had no desire to become a Catholic or anything (and still don't). It was all about her. Who was she?

I started reading books about Mary and found it interesting that in the history of Catholicism there have been precious few Jesus sightings, but enormous numbers of Mary sightings (and she appears in the race of the people who see her). People love her!

As I read, it reminded me that the environmental and organic movement as well as religion use fear to manage their adherents. If you sin, you are going to hell. If you marry someone from a different faith, you will be banished. If you have sex outside of the bounds we set, you will be stoned to death. No religion was exempt from this fear-based intimidation. Somehow I hadn't fully seen this before.

But then there was Mary. She would kiss it and make it better. Mary, as the popular T-shirt slogan states, became my "home-girl." Long before *The Da Vinci Code* became a runaway best seller, scholars and writers had been writing about her. Through them and my own inner explorations, I discovered her long and illustrious tradition, one that had begun well before written history and way before she was declared a virgin by the Catholic Church. I then read a book called *Sacred Pleasure* by Riane Eisler, which explored how ancient, female-based religions viewed pleasure seeking as an act of worship. And that was it. Before I knew it, I'd found lots of other "pleasure revolutionaries" throughout history who had walked the path before me and cleared the way. I learned a third lesson: Pleasure is an ancient, sacred path.

With that, I tripped, stumbled, and fell for good. I was now permanently and forever on the path of pleasure. And I will not turn back.

What does Maya have to do with all of this? In many ways, my daughter was my catalyst, my reason for it all: my search, my frustration with society and religion, my determination to find answers. When I was nineteen and alone in a dorm room, realizing I was pregnant; realizing that many in my family and my boyfriend wanted me to have an abortion; realizing that I would probably be shunned by the people I knew (after all, it was 1981—upper-class white girls having kids out of wedlock just wasn't done back then—at least publicly); realizing that my future was in my own hands; I trusted my heart and soul. I listened to the tiny voice inside of me that said, "I am terrified, but I do not want to have an abortion. Everything happens for a reason—I don't know why it is right now but I'll find out some day. God doesn't give you challenges you can't handle—I am going to keep this baby because I don't want to live with the regret of what might have been." I realized the true meaning of "choice"; having a child at such a young age wasn't for everyone, nor should it be, but this was my path.

And so I kept my baby. Now she's my best friend. We both are tripping and stumbling along this path of pleasure and laughing at our head-bonks and stupid mistakes . . . and always stopping to watch Thursday night TV. We comfort each other through our crying fits and depressive episodes.

Pleasure isn't really about happiness or sadness. Of course, the path of pleasure is bound to lead to more happiness. Still, happiness is fleeting. Bad days and moods are inevitable, and often monthly. But pleasure is something you can keep with you and draw on in good times and bad. Those moments of self-discovery can strike you even when you're down, if you invite them to, and we've found that pleasure is always the result. Pleasure is a path of hope and optimism, belief in love and, yes, romance! It's a path that leads to happy endings and true love, but it's up to each of us to create it. We'll let you know what's worked for us. But ultimately the journey is yours to take and create. And the pleasure is yours, too.

DRIVING DOWN THE HIGHWAY OF PLEASURE—MAYA

According to some people, I should be a total screwup. I lived with my single mother and had no biological father figure. I watched MTV and movies featuring nudity and sex at a young and impressionable age. I learned and used quite a few curse words at the age of four. I never made my bed. I played with Barbies. And although I had lots of cousins and aunts and uncles and grandparents around— all of whom adored me—the center of my universe was always my mom and I. And the strong bond between us is part of the reason I think I turned out OK.

Because it was most often just the two of us, we had to spend time together and love each other and become friends. All in all, we had (and have) lots of good times together. We share music (although when I borrow CDs I rarely give them back); we go to movies together; we talk about books we read. She gave me all her old Barbie clothes. We spent Saturdays at work—she had her desk, and I had mine in a corner of her office. We drove all over town on endless rounds of errands. For a while, we lived in a one-bedroom basement apartment in Washington, D.C. We talk on the phone every single day, sometimes twice.

But liberal as my mum is and was about bedtimes, sex, and stuff like that, she also was overprotective. I wasn't allowed to cross the street by myself until I was around eleven. I was forbidden to drive by myself until I was almost eighteen. Eventually, after all the pain and drama and oppression, I finally was allowed to take the car out. And, damn, was it good. It felt like life really began for me when I learned to drive. One of my favorite things to do is drive on the highway with the music really, really loud, singing along, with happy tears in my eyes. Something about that makes me feel the glory and magic of the universe to an insane degree. I guess it's what really religious people get out of church.

Ours wasn't a religious home. I was baptized at the age of two. My mother's rationale was, "Just in case. It couldn't hurt." I remember sitting in my eighth grade religion class, wondering how people could worship a God that seemed boring and petty. (I was in a nondenominational private school, so we spent equal time on the "big five"—Christianity, Judaism, Islam, Hinduism, Buddhism). Yet, all religions intrigued me. I was encouraged to learn about them without predetermined expectations of what I should believe, so, in high school, I thought of myself as shopping for a religion because I felt the urge to be spiritually connected to the universe. I would try one on and see if it fit. And none of them did. Some demanded that I renounce meat. Ha! All of them had body issues. I did not, perhaps because bodies were never treated as shameful in our house, and I was allowed to watch a movie with sex in it before I was allowed to watch anything violent. A lot of them talked about my inherent and eternal flaws, which my heart rebelled against. All in all, I found them to be a little tight in the crotch. I did, however, notice the Virgin Mary prayer on the refrigerator and my mother's growing collection of Marys. Maybe I didn't need a "pants" religion; maybe I needed a skirt.

A high school English teacher of mine said that everyone has "One Book" that changes the way they see the world. She claimed that if we read anything by Ayn Rand, then that would be The One. I had already read them, but at the time, I still considered myself searching for That Book. And while I no longer subscribe to that notion, a certain book did dramatically change the way I saw the world. It was *The Templar Revelation* by Lynn Picknett and Clive Prince, which my mom gave me when I came home for winter break my first year of college, saying, "You have to read this." I sat on the couch of our hard-core Catholic relatives' house that holiday and read about the secret life of Jesus Christ and Mary Magdalene. More importantly, I discovered ancient goddess worship for the first time and a new perspective on history, religion, and the world. Finally, I was finding, if not a religion, at least a spiritual outlet that worked for me—where sex was a powerful creative way of worship;

where it was not only okay to be a girl, but exalted; where being human was the same thing as being divine.

This book also prompted conversations between my mother and me, where we would ask, "Why don't people know this?" Of course, since publication of *The Da Vinci Code*, millions of people have some of the information. But our conversations, with that question as the refrain, are one of the reasons we decided to write this book.

All this couldn't have come at a better time for me. I needed a grander context in which to understand my life, and that book had started me on the path to finding it. I had just started college and all of a sudden had to deal with boys and sex, new friends and alcohol, and a freedom I had never known before. I had thought I wouldn't be able to have a normal relationship with boys because I never had a father figure. I got over that one. I didn't have guilt issues regarding sex, but I had to figure out (through trial and error) what sex meant to me, and what kind of sex I wanted to be having. My social life had revolved around tequila shots (we have since parted ways). I did have some kickass girlfriends, thank goodness. But in spite of some good moments, I hated my life at college. I constantly felt suffocated. One night I had to get out of the commotion in my dorm room to be alone and think and had nowhere to go. I ended up on the steps of the library with my journal and Walkman. People looked at me funny, but I didn't care. I wrote about wishing I was in a café somewhere in a big city.

That was one of my first conscious pleasure moments—and I simply had to prolong it. I had listened to the quiet of my heart, and was finally of an age where I could take action. I found a summer program in Paris and took off to live the best six consecutive weeks of my life so far. In Paris, for the first time ever, I walked alone down the cobblestone streets and laughed at the sheer joy of being alive and doing something so simple that was so perfect. I spent hours alone in cafés writing. I had a little love affair. I made friends. I spent hours in the Louvre looking for what I read about in *The Templar Revelation*. I found statues and paintings of beautiful women. I sauntered through outdoor markets. I went shopping. All in all, I lived quite well. I was deliriously happy.

Then I had to return to college in the fall. Coming from Paris back to a small town in Connecticut was like a hangover that wouldn't end. I woke up crying. I took long drives through the countryside, playing music really loud, trying to figure out what I needed to do to fall in love with life again. After many of these trips I decided I had to move to New York City.

During the drive to my new school, I had an unforgettable moment of panic. I was safely in the backseat with my parents up front, and suddenly we were in loud, chaotic, colorful Chinatown driving toward my new dorm. I had never seen this part of the city. I suddenly had the thought that I'd played a practical joke on myself, and that it had gone too far. And everyone else had fallen for it, too. Did I really want this freedom? What had I gotten myself into? But there was no going back.

And, thank goodness for that, because I fell in love with life again. Growing up with my overprotective mother, I still get excited about going out and walking around the city all by myself without asking permission. I stay out late—just because I can. I love having so many choices that it's almost a burden. I love that when I first arrived in Chinatown that January day I had very little but suitcases and hope, and two years later I have a full life that I created all by myself.

At first I had maybe two friends, so I threw myself into my schoolwork. I ended up majoring in Women & Fiction. My mother insisted I couldn't legitimately accept that degree without reading a romance novel. After all, they are written by women for women about women. In the name of research, I read one and then another and another, as well as all those ancient goddess history books. And I started to wonder how I could apply all this rich stuff to my real life.

In high school I earned the nickname "The Mankiller," which had stuck through the beginning of college. But then I realized I didn't want to be that kind of girl—one that would flirt but never let her heart open up and love. But I also didn't know who I wanted to turn myself into, especially in relationships with boys. I had grown up on Madonna and the idea of periodic reinvention of oneself. So I created a mantra for myself: Books before Boys. I went on strike, at least until I had met a good man. And when I did find one, I had finally gotten to the point where I was ready and willing to be in a relationship. Ours may not be a romance-novel kind of love, and it certainly has its ups and downs, but it's pretty darn close.

Throughout all of this, my mom and I talked on the phone every day, even when I was in Europe. We were reading the same books and, like partnering detectives, we shared notes and thoughts. We thought and talked about the lives we wanted to live, and knew we wanted them to be happy, and satisfying, and pleasurable. With the books on history, religion, sex, and romance novels, we realized that we—and all women—not only deserved pleasure, but also had the capacity to give it to themselves. It was up to us to create it. So we did. Somewhere in all our conversations we decided to write a book about what we were reading, thinking, and talking about. I cannot remember when we decided this, or when we started, or what life was like before it began to take shape. It just seems always to have been present in our lives in some form or another.

But I do remember being eight years old, riding shotgun in the car with my mom, both of us singing along to Madonna's "Like a Prayer" on the radio. Looking back now, I remember, vaguely, that the world had a temper fit because the video showed a woman mixing sexuality and passion, power and religion without guilt or shame and above all, in a fun way. My mom and I didn't bat an eyelash at all that—we just sang along. Little did we know that years later we would be rediscovering how to do that in our own lives. And, of course, having fun along the way.

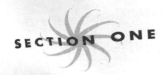

What's *Your* Pleasure? Find Your True Self

THE JOURNEY TOWARDS PLEASURE STARTS INSIDE OF YOU, and in knowing who you are and what you want—what *your* pleasure is. But because life is in a constant state of change and movement, finding your true self is an ongoing process. To start a revolution in your own life you need to figure out who you are *now*, at this special, specific moment in time. Where did you wake up this morning and what were your first thoughts? Are you looking forward to your day with excitement or dread? Why do you feel guilty about some things and not others? Do you need more pleasure in your life? What in your life has led you to this place where you are now? Where do you really want to go next?

Before you can truly understand your world, your life, and your relationships you must at least try to understand yourself and what truly gives *you* joy and satisfaction. You may know exactly what this is, already, or like many women, you may have become so busy with family or work that your own individual needs have gotten submerged by others.

But finding yourself is not a chore. In our process in this book, there will be no fasting or climbs to caves in search of some unbathed guru. The only guru you need is right inside of you. The only tools you need are time, space, and a slightly open mind—these are the greatest gifts that only you can give to yourself. And pleasure is the reward.

Do you need more pleasure in your life?

TAKE THIS QUIZ TO FIND OUT YOUR PLEASURE PERSONALITY

1. I feel guilty for:
   - a. everything
   - b. feeling guilty
   - c. a few things, like eating too many desserts
   - d. nothing

2. In my everyday life, I put my own needs:
   - a. what needs?
   - b. last
   - c. before the pets, but after the kids and husband
   - d. first

3. I get massages:
   - a. never. I don't let strangers touch my body.
   - b. rarely
   - c. when I need it, or can afford it
   - d. regularly

4. When I find myself alone, I:
   - a. freak out and call somebody
   - b. clean the house or watch TV
   - c. read a book or take a nap
   - d. am thrilled with the possibilities

5. I see exercise as:
   - a. a necessary evil
   - b. an unnecessary evil
   - c. time for me
   - d. a form of play that keeps me balanced

ily is:

hem

:

ife

ple

r is:
of your business

and clean
y, clean, and comfortable

shop, I:
lways find the least expensive choice
enjoy bargain hunting, but splurge occasionally
. go for quality over quantity
d. buy it if I love it (if I can afford it)

here is a rule I don't like, I:
a. follow it anyway
b. tolerate it
c. occasionally break it
d. disregard it

9. Love is:
a. a fairytale fantasy
b. hard
c. sweet
d. what makes the world go round

6. Dinner is~

4

13. My relationship with my fam
    a. a strained obligation
    b. tense, but I ignore t
    c. fine
    d. hysterically fun

14. When I get depressed,
    a. suffer through i
    b. take a pill
    c. go for a walk
    d. examine my

8. Cho
    a.
    b. 1
    c. an
    d. an e~

15. My body is:
    a. a burden
    b. a tool
    c. my body
    d. my tem

9. My life is:
    a. depressing
    b. predictable
    c. occasionally e~
    d. an adventure

16. My underwe~
    a. none
    b. clea~
    c. sexy
    d. se~

10. Romance novels are:
    a. trash
    b. formulaic and insulting
    c. my embarrassing secret
    d. my delightful escape

17. When I
    a.
    b.
    c

11. When I see other people having fun ~
    a. feel angry
    b. feel jealous
    c. feel competitive
    d. feel happy

18. If t

12. For vacations, I like to:
    a. stay with family
    b. go to the same place every year
    c. stay in hotels I'm familiar with
    d. go places I've never been before

1

20. I think women:
      a. belong in the home
      b. shouldn't try to compete with men
      c. are fun to hang around with
      d. are powerful and can change the world

If you got mostly:

As: You are a **Pleasure Puritan.** You need pleasure so badly it hurts to watch. With a little bit of an open mind and an open heart, your whole life can blossom if you just let it.

Bs: You are a **Pleasure Pincher.** You are in need of a pleasure transfusion. It's not fatal, but it could be if you don't start looking for more pleasure right now. The capacity for more pleasure is within you.

Cs: You are a **Pleasure Adventuress.** You go, girl! You are on the right path and have tasted some of the delights of pleasure. Keep going, you are almost to the magic palace!

Ds: You are a **Pleasure Revolutionary.** Congratulations! You are a model for other women to follow, but we know that's not why you do it. You love pleasure. You love life. And people love being with you because your pleasure is contagious. Keep on spreading the love.

The Goddess

To get to the root of female pleasure we want to tell you the story of women's history.

In the beginning, before Adam and Eve, before Abraham, Jesus, and Mohammed, before Buddha, there was a woman. Call her the first Mother, or the Goddess. In fact, she had many, many names. For example, in the Old Testament, she is called Astarte, Queen of Heaven. But her name doesn't really matter because she was worshipped practically everywhere—for she represented the abundance, fertility, and beauty of nature.

This sacred female principle was known to have three faces. Her first face, or manifestation, was that of the Virgin. Her other faces were Mother and Crone, or elderly wise woman.

Back in the olden days "virgin" didn't mean what we think of now (sexual virtue intact). Back then, the word virgin meant, simply, "unmarried." According to *The Woman's Encyclopedia of Myths and Secrets*, the priestesses of Ishtar, Asherah, or Aphrodite were known as "Holy Virgins" even though they had sex as part of the rituals of worship. These priestesses were the original "brides" of God, and their offspring were considered "virgin-born."

Several thousand years ago, however, this female Goddess, her culture and followers, were overthrown by an invasion of people who worshipped a male God. These people set up their God to rule over the Goddess, yet she continued to be worshipped, often hidden in plain sight. In one manifestation, the Goddess became the Virgin Mary, "Queen of Heaven," who gave birth to the Son of God. She is also the lady of the lake, and present anywhere there is a sacred spring or well (water is considered her "blood"). The Goddess is also the young, beautiful princess of fairy tales, struggling to find her prince and always receiving the help of nature along the way. She is Aphrodite, the Greek goddess of love. In ancient Rome, she was Venus, and was represented by the sea. The Goddess provides salvation with the power of her love.

She is the beginning of our history, and she holds the roots to the mystery of pleasure.

CHAPTER 1

Go to Your Room

Pleasure starts in the quiet
of your own heart

THE PLEASURE OF SUNDAYS—MARIA

My favorite moment of a regular week is Sunday morning. My husband Lou, daughter Eve, our dog Pippa, and I have all read the local paper and the *New York Times* together. I've had a few cups of strong, black coffee. It's still too early for Maya to call me from New York. Lou gathers Eve and together off they go to church.

Exhale! I've got two glorious hours to myself!

I love my family dearly, truly I do. But there is something about being alone in my own home that is precious and even essential to my sanity. For two fabulous hours I can do whatever I want. I can eat what I want without asking what anyone else wants and making it for them. I can decide simply to read or write without having to share my space with a jumping, dancing (adorable) kid, chewing dog, or the static of sports radio, which my husband inexplicably finds most appealing.

After the dust of their leaving settles and I send the dog outside to play, I can take stock: Of the house—which is usually a total disaster area. Of my life—which usually needs a massive organizing list-fest. Of my body—which usually needs some sort of physical release. But most important, of my soul—which in the course of my frenzied week usually gets lost. On Sunday morning, while being alone, I manage to find Me again.

I guess that's why some people go to church. It's why I stay home.

I developed my appreciation for being alone in my room early. I was the fourth of five children. My oldest sister, Heather, was a classic eldest sibling—second mother and in charge of everything and everybody. My second oldest sister, Heidi, was quietly squeezed between her older sister and our brother, David, the first son and "heir," who was the center of attention from a very early age. Then there was me and after me my younger brother, Anthony, who was hyperactive, and all boy.

My mother was a force of nature. When she was happy, she was very happy, and when she was sad, she was very sad. Often she was ill, and many times she felt underappreciated. And my father, when he wasn't working or traveling, was lost in his own private universe, otherwise known as "the study." My mother will be the first to tell you that a lot of her frustration came from my father. He wanted a wife who didn't work (but she did—often without pay). He wanted dinner on the table every night at five-thirty, and would often bring business guests without warning. He preferred quiet nights at home, while she would rather have gone out every night dancing. I got my rebellious nature from my mother, I think, and my studiousness from my father.

Being alone in my room seemed to be the only place where I had space to find myself. Space to be ME.

When I was really little I would lie on my bed with my fuzzy golden blanket, dreaming that its folds and ripples around my legs were the sand dunes of the great Sahara desert. I was riding on my camel searching for an oasis, and perhaps stumbling on a lost civilization. I think I was supposed to be taking a nap, but I was alone in my room and happier than usual.

A few years later, while my mother was downstairs crying that no one appreciated her (and my "but I love you, Mommy" wasn't enough), I would pretend that I was a princess and my room was my kingdom, Camelot, and I was King Arthur and Guinevere *and* the dashing, handsome Sir Lancelot. At other times, I was a detective, solving the mystery of the universe right next to Nancy Drew and Ned Nickerson. More often, I was an orphaned eccentric like Pippi, who ate without utensils and didn't have to worry about cleaning up after myself. That fantasy lasted until my mother would start shrieking at the top of her lungs about what a pig I was and I had to clean up my room immediately "or ELSE!" Then I turned into Cinderella.

When I was a teenager, my room became a sanctuary from the crazy, confusing world, and my family. I was an artist, painting my masterpieces and smoking in the bathroom. I was writing great stories on my dusty, inky old typewriter (yes, it was before computers). I was a desirable, fiercely independent hoyden reading romance novels and waiting for a *real* man to come across my path rather than the stupid boys I knew. With my scratchy turntable (this was also before CDs and even cassette tapes), I was transported to a land where parents got along, siblings didn't make fun of and demean their beloved sister, and friends were faithful and true. It may have been the marijuana I smoked that was transporting me, but I could dream about making a future that was better than my present. I could dream about being and becoming anything. Because no one was around to tell me otherwise.

I used fantasy and my imagination to get through some pretty difficult times. Years later, when I read *Reviving Ophelia*, when Maya was a teenager spending lots of time alone in her room, I was reassured to learn that some of the strongest, best, most successful women did the very same thing.

How can you ever know who you really are without being in a place where no one else is telling you who you are or who you aren't— or at the very least *not* telling you what to do? You need a safe place to explore, create, discover, uncover, reflect, revise, and just plain enjoy being who you are. You have to take the time to figure out what gives you pleasure or what gives you pain, and sort through what has happened to you and why.

Women—at least of my generation and older—were often raised to be constantly focused on other people's needs, emotions, and hunger level. I was told through myriad sources (often at church) to put other people's needs before my own. I learned to feel that the greatest sin a woman could commit was to be selfish. And that all other sins stem from that. But all around me were women, like my mother and grandmothers, who were furious at everyone almost all the time, because they had had to put others' needs before their own. They were supposed to know what others wanted as well as needed without asking, and to deliver without expecting anything in return.

Recently, my mother and I were talking about the difficult times she had when I was young. When I was three she was terribly depressed and drinking a lot due to her unexpected pregnancy with her fifth child. After he was born, she developed myocarditis (an infection of the lining of the heart). Just when she recovered from that, she got spinal meningitis. Her doctor said she'd never walk again (although it's hard to keep up with her now!). I asked her why she thought she had suffered from so many health problems. She answered: "I was giving and giving to everyone but myself. I had lost my soul."

So here I am. It's Sunday morning. This is my time. If I feel up to it, I try to clean off the kitchen table—which seems to be the receptacle of all our flotsam and jetsam. (And it never fails that the first thing my husband does when he walks in after church is put the church bulletin right on it—as if I cleaned it just for him!) Sometimes I read. Sometimes I write. Sometimes I make lists. Sometimes I listen to music or sing and other times I simply enjoy the silence.

But I always, always feel better. So when little Eve comes running in the house and jumps into my arms, I am truly ready to be Mom again. When Lou comes in and puts his church bulletin on the table, I am ready to be his wife again—without resentment. When the phone rings and it's Maya telling me all about work last night, I'm ready to listen. When I tackle that pile of work, I am ready to be a business-woman again.

And whatever I or we decide to do the rest of the day, whether it's food shopping, working, or just plain living . . . I know that I am ME again.

A BED/OFFICE/DINING/LIVING ROOM
OF MY OWN—MAYA

*B*eing alone in your room, like most things in life, is what you make of it. It can seem like a prison, or it can be a refuge, depending on how you look at it. For me, my room is a haven: the place I go when the rest of the world is too much to handle, or when I am feeling sad, or when I am mentally tired. There I sit around day-

…eaming, or drawing, or writing, or just looking out the window. As a child and a teenager, everything felt better when I was alone in my room. I could walk through the door and know that it was My Place, and this was My Time for Myself.

Living in college dorms with dozens of roommates made "alone time" nearly unattainable, and therefore priceless. Sometimes I would skip class to sit around in the room when I knew my roommate wouldn't be there. I justified it with a line from Rumi, a thirteenth century poet: "A little while alone in your room will prove more valuable than anything else that could ever be given to you." For a twenty-four-hour period when I was particularly blessed, I found myself in a hotel room in the middle of a blizzard, deliciously alone except for the occasional room service delivery. I read Virginia Woolf's *A Room of One's Own* and stared out at the snowy New York City streets, fantasizing about being a writer, living in my own apartment. All by myself.

In my room was where I imagined things. And these fantasies sort of came true. But what I am finding out, that I did not expect, is that there is an art to being alone in one's room, and alone with oneself and actually enjoying it. Because now, in real life and not in my imagination, I am a writer, living alone, and it is not as perfect as I had imagined.

For example, I live in a studio apartment (a "bed-sitting-room" as Virginia Woolf called it). When my friends come over, we joke, "let's move to the living room" and we move to the couch. "Hold on, I have to get something from my bedroom," I say, taking two steps and I'm already there. My desk by the window has become my office. Every morning, after coffee and the paper, I say, "OK, time to go to work," and I'm already there. Even though I really like to write, since I am getting paid for it, it qualifies as work. And working within sight of one's bed is *really* hard. The plus side is that I have a really short commute; the down side is that I have days when I go stir-crazy. I'm not complaining, but I have found out that time to myself alone in my room requires more ingredients than just myself and an empty room.

Every Sunday, I tell myself that I don't have to work. My desk is right there, with my computer and books I should read for research.

But I don't do it; I give myself a day off from obligations. And somehow it just feels better, different. It's still me, in the same room, day after day. But it's the attitude I bring; it's what I make of it. On Sundays, my apartment is just my room, where I can putter around, not really doing anything; on Monday morning, it becomes an office again.

I was at the dentist the other day, and as the lady worked on my teeth she talked about her daughter who was home from college and was spending hours quietly alone in her room. Getting curious, her mother knocked on the door to ask what she was doing. "Just playing," was the reply. I couldn't reply, because I had a mouth full of dental tools, but I thought how I understood exactly, and had done the same things many, many times. I lock myself in my room, turn off the cell phone, and I don't really do anything. I just hang out and catch up on quality time with myself.

DO IT: BE ALONE IN YOUR ROOM FOR
TWO UNINTERRUPTED HOURS

You can do this one. It's easy! Especially if you already live alone. If you don't, you'll have to think of a way to arrange some solitude.

Going to your room alone while others are in the house is great. But it's not as great as if you are alone in the whole house or apartment. That way, if you decide to sing at the top of your lungs, no one rolls his or her eyes or has fodder for future teasing. Your goal is to be in a space where you can be completely uninhibited. Maybe you even need to go to a hotel for a night by yourself to get it. That works, too.

Do not, under any circumstances, start cleaning. We women tend to clean compulsively, often as an excuse for not doing other, more productive things. If your room or your house is a mess, sit and think and meditate in your space as to why it is such a mess, and ask for inspiration into more permanent solutions. For instance, maybe what you really need to do is a complete reorganization, or move, or set up new house rules. Being alone is not about avoiding thinking about being alone. It's about thinking about you, you, you.

LIST: TOP TEN THINGS TO DO ALONE IN YOUR ROOM

Write—It can be anything. An easy place to start is just venting with a pen and paper. Don't even bother with the pressure of a journal or diary. Scraps of paper or a tablet will do.

Draw—What would your dream house look like? Your ideal wardrobe? Try a doodle or two. What you end up doodling when you are not really focusing is a window into your subconscious, and perhaps into what you want.

Sleep—A nap is the greatest necessity disguised as a luxury. If you are tired and cranky, it's hard to be or do anything else.

Sing—Along with the radio, or just by yourself.

Make lists—Of things you have to do—anticipating the satisfaction of crossing it out—and of things you've always wanted to do, own. or experience.

Dream—Pure fun. Allow yourself to fantasize about whatever your heart desires. Love, sex, wealth, success, freedom, travel. In your dreams there are no limits and no credit card bills, either.

Read—Anything that you become immersed in will do. But you might want to stay away from stressful books, or anything with an unhappy ending. A romance novel should keep you absorbed for a few hours. Get lost in one and see what it feels like to expect a happy ending.

Dance—It's fun, and it's exercise. And if you do it right to really loud music you can get into a trance and really feel the bliss.

Pamper yourself—Hot baths, do your nails . . . figure out what makes you feel good. Then do it.

Explore your body—We women are so busy checking our faces or teeth in the mirror that we often forget the rest of our body. We know one woman who was so concerned about her puffy and wrinkled eyes that she went in for an eye lift before she realized she had a giant melanoma on the bottom of her foot. Take a good look at your whole body. Try to appreciate it and enjoy it. Don't be afraid to touch yourself, either. *Tirade Alert!* By the way, did you know that until around 1712 masturbation was not even considered sinful? But then a doctor wrote a book called: *Onania; or, The Heinous Sin of Self Pollution, and all its Frightful Consequences, in both SEXES Considered, with Spiritual and Physical Advice to those who have already injured themselves by this abominable practice*. It became a global best seller, as did his "cure" of "Strengthening Tincture" and "Prolific Powder." (See *Solitary Sex*, by Thomas W. Laqueur.) Onan is the guy from the Old Testament who is blamed for making "spilling his seed" a sin. Historians who have looked at the original versions of the Bible realized that Onan's real sin was that he refused to impregnate his dead brother's wife and "perform the duty of a brother-in-law to her; raise up offspring for your brother." The actual story, Genesis 38:9 continues: "But since Onan knew that the offspring would not be his, he spilled his semen on the ground whenever he went in to his brother's wife, so that he would not give offspring to his brother." God killed Onan for that, not for masturbating. Even in medieval times, it was a greater sin to have hot, passionate sex in a nonmissionary position with your own spouse than it was to "spill seed."

IN HER OWN VOICE: GEORGIA O'KEEFFE

"I've been lucky. Maybe because I've taken hold of anything that came along that I've wanted. . . . But life is like a knife. On this knife I might fall off on either side. But I'd walk it again. So what—what if you do fall off? I'd rather be doing something I really *wanted* to do."

"If I can't work by myself for a year with no stimulus other than what I can find in books, distant friends, and my own fun in living, then I'm not worth much."

On painting giant flowers: "It just amused me."

PLEASURE REVOLUTIONARY: GEORGIA O'KEEFFE

Virginia Woolf coined the phrase "a woman needs five hundred pounds a year and a room of one's own," but it took a woman like Georgia O'Keeffe to show the world what a little "alone time" could bring. She is one of only a handful of female painters on a par with men in the art world. Impressionist Mary Cassatt is equally famous, but for paintings of a woman's domain—motherhood. One of the few female painters who is internationally recognized, O'Keeffe's paintings have a distinct style that is unequaled. And she certainly spent time alone in her room.

At twelve years old, she knew she wanted to be a painter. Her parents never approved of "Georgia's crazy notions." But she educated herself in the art of her time. After years of painting to please other people she became disgusted with her own work. "There wasn't anything to please myself and I thought it was pretty dull. So I put it all away and started over again," she said.

When O'Keeffe was just out of college she spent a year in Texas teaching. During the nights, she "sat on the floor and worked against the closet door" in her room, drawing shapes she says she could only see in her head. Eventually, O'Keeffe and her paintings had to leave her bedroom. They all ended up in Alfred Stieglitz's New York City gallery, 192, after a friend of O'Keeffe's secretly sent her paintings there.

O'Keeffe and Stieglitz first met about her work and became one of the greatest love stories of all time. Their initial encounter was quite heated because O'Keeffe was furious that Stieglitz was showing her paintings without her permission. She got over it. After years of letter writing, and artistically inspiring and supporting each other, they married, and each continued to pursue his and her art. Considered the father of modern photography, Stieglitz worshipped O'Keeffe with his camera, leaving perhaps the largest photographic documentation of any woman in history.

In an interview, Georgia O'Keeffe recounts what it was like hanging out with Stieglitz and other artists. "Stieglitz had to have people around him," she said. "I find people very difficult. And when I couldn't take it I'd go into my room and shut the door." Not even Alfred was allowed into her room when she was painting.

Some of the time she lived in New York City with Stieglitz and a few million other people, or she stayed at Lake George in a house with more than twenty members of her family. Every once in a while she would take off for New Mexico, where she lived off and on for a few years, eventually settling there permanently. Going out West was key to her creativity. "When I got to New Mexico, that was mine. It fitted to me exactly. . . . I feel like myself. And I like it." An interviewer mentioned how nice it was of Stieglitz to let her go to New Mexico every summer. "Well, listen," she laughs, "he didn't let me go, I just went . . . I had to go."

She painted bones because they pleased her. She painted giant flowers because they amused her. She lived her life exactly as she wanted to. And she became a successful artist, a painter, just like she knew she would be when she was alone in her room at age twelve.

CHAPTER 2

Use Your Fear as Your Guide

Pleasure may seem scary at first,
but it doesn't bite

FACING MY FAUX FEARS—MARIA

There are two kinds of fear: real fear and faux fear. Real fear includes all the truly bad stuff: fear of terrible things happening to your family, fear of lions, tigers, and bears, fear of dark alleys and dangerous ex-boyfriends, and the biggie: fear of death. I have a healthy, respectful fear of death, having grieved for two old grandmothers, a brother who died suddenly of AIDS in 1985, and my father who died even more suddenly in a car crash in Moscow in 1990. I'm not as afraid of my own death (as long as it's fairly quick and unexpected) as I am of the loss of precious people in my life. I think most of us feel that way. But I'm not going to dwell on death here. It's a mystery I am not going to solve today.

The fear I want to talk to you about in this chapter is real, but kind of like a paper tiger. Once you walk through it, you realize it wasn't that scary at all: it's what I call faux fear. One of the most common faux fears is fear of what other people will think. That is what I was most afraid of when I decided to keep my baby when I was nineteen. What will everyone think? They will know I had sex . . . shame on me! Later

I realized the real thing to be afraid of is giving birth. It hurts! I think it took me fifteen years to get over the fear of childbirth in order to have Eve . . . but I'm so glad I did (plus, she arrived while I was under complete general anesthesia).

Another really awful faux fear that gets a lot of people, including me sometimes, is the fear of trying new things. What if I don't like it or it tastes really bad? I draw the line at things like sea urchin and head cheese (which has more to do with texture than principle), but I tried foie gras and liver (by accident) and can honestly say I don't care for them.

The fear of new things includes fear of new experiences. Once, a friend of mine had really bad cancer. My yoga teacher at the time suggested I do a special Hindu prayer ceremony for him, even though my friend wasn't Hindu. I thought to myself, "Oh what the heck, it can't hurt." My teacher arranged for the ceremony, but while I was waiting for it to begin I felt this terror—as if something evil would happen if I stayed, as if it was wrong of me to dabble in someone else's faith. But I was stuck, and the priests showed up, looking kind of cute with sneakers on under their white robes. We had brought them big bars of chocolate as thanks. I didn't understand a word of the ceremony, but it included flower petals, incense, oil, seeds—it was a sensual feast and I felt as if I had ventured into another world. I had. I was sent home with a bucket of holy water and carnation blossoms for my friend to sprinkle around his home, which he did.

I had a truly lovely experience. I had sat through my faux fear and I did not convert to Hinduism. I did not get brainwashed into an ashram cult. Best of all, my friend recovered fully from his cancer—whether because of the ceremony or not, we will never know.

Fear of public speaking is a notoriously common fear. Some surveys rank it as even higher than fear of death! Unfortunately or fortunately I have to do a lot of public speaking in my job. I can't hide behind my fear. But I can say this is one fear that lessens the more you fight it and do the speaking. I've had some truly awful things happen to me while speaking in public—so I'm just happy if I don't fall on stage or vomit (although people seem to survive that, too). When I was giving out an award at a trade conference, I was the last speaker before lunch and the previous speaker had gone over her time by a half hour. Even though my presentation was only five minutes, between the time I got up to the podium and when I handed out the award, eight thousand people had gotten up and left the room. The only people left were the award recipient and a few co-workers. I survived.

So now, whenever I feel fear I analyze it. Is it real or faux? If I'm on a plane I remember that the odds of something bad happening are quite low. If my family or I am in any physical danger, I take precautions and trust my instincts—I try to differentiate fear and instinct so that I am not using my "instincts" as a reason not to do something. For example, if I am traveling to a foreign city, my fear might be telling me to stay in the hotel room or something scary might happen out there. But I know it's important to go out anyway. Once I am out, I use my common sense to guide me in the right direction and away from dark scary streets or frightening neighborhoods.

When in doubt, I pray for protection. But if it's just the curtain of fear, the paper tiger, the faux fear, I let myself feel it, recognize it for what it is, face it head on, and walk right through. And I've always found a whole new world on the other side. And in that new world, pleasure lives.

A LIFE LIVED IN FEAR IS A LIFE HALF LIVED—MAYA

After months of meetings and conference calls and conversations about pleasure and love and romance novels and all the ingredients of this book, our agent, Linda, said she hadn't read a romance novel yet. And was afraid to.

"But, how can this be?" I asked, as if she had just said she thought breathing was a waste of time.

"I guess I'm just afraid that once I start I won't be able to stop," she replied.

"Oh, Linda, I was there once, too. You'll get over it," I said in the voice my mother uses when I declare I want to do something ridiculous, like get my nose pierced. "Oh, Maya. You'll get over it." (I did get over the desire, thankfully, before I got it done.)

When my mom first started reading romance novels, during my junior year of college, I made fun of her for it. I should have known better. Whenever I make fun of her for something, I find myself obsessed and devoted to that very same thing within months. So I scoffed and dissed but she kept reading and trying to get me to read them, too.

"But Mom," I whined, "I cannot. I have to read *Ulysses* and *Madame Bovary* for school!" I was afraid that I would love romance novels so much that the classics would become unbearable, I wouldn't be able to read anything else again, and I would fail out of school with nothing to comfort me but a stack of mass market paperbacks.

But my mom gave me a reason to read romances with which I could not argue: research. My major was women in literature—as writers and characters. Mom convinced me that there was no legitimate way for me to receive my degree if I didn't read the most popular and profitable books in the world, written by women and for women. Naturally, no college course I had come across had a romance novel on the syllabus; not even the class I took about love in literature. "All right, you have a point," I said grudgingly. "Send me a reading list."

The list had books like *Pride and Prejudice* and *The Natural History of the Romance Novel,* along with some strongly recommended paperbacks, like *Shanna,* by Kathleen Woodiwiss. I tried, but we didn't click. And then one day I picked up *The Flame and the Flower*. And I have never looked back.

I added a romance novel to my colloquium book list, right between *Ulysses* and *Madame Bovary*. My professors were tolerant and intrigued, although against their better judgment, I could tell. I compared and contrasted: the happy with the sad, the respected with the bad reputation. I got my degree. And I kept reading romance novels.

They were addicting, they were fun, they made me happy, and as far as I could tell, they didn't have any negative side effects. Sure, I now had high standards for what I looked for in a man, but that actually worked out for the better. When I started reading romance novels, a certain boy laughed and scoffed and said I was smarter than that. We didn't work out. And while I was wandering around, paperback in my handbag and a new idea of love in my little heart—a love where men and women could be themselves and evolve and overcame obstacles and love triumphed over everything—I met another boy. One who had the build of romance novel hero, and one who didn't laugh at me when I went on at length about dukes and ballrooms. We've been together for a year now, and I think that that is due in part to a faith in love and newfound role models in heroines that don't punk out when the honeymoon phase is over.

I have always loved a movie called *Strictly Ballroom*. It's a romantic comedy, which is basically very similar to a romance novel, about a very handsome guy who is a ballroom dancer, but keeps dancing his own invented steps in competitions. Everyone thinks he's crazy and tries to stop him, except for the heroine, of course. The recurring theme of this movie is that "A life lived in fear is a life half lived." If he doesn't dance the way his heart tells him to, he will live a life in fear, like his father before him. He will not truly live. Eventually, he finds the right partner, who is also the right girl, and they dance their new steps, winning the competition and the respect of those who had been against them. Like every romance novel, it had a happy ending.

"A life lived in fear is a life half lived" is a lovely mantra, and I repeat it to myself whenever I am afraid of something that I know I have to face. It gives me the strength to at least try to overcome my fear. And if this idea is illustrated anywhere, it is in a romance novel. Pirates, would-be rapists, kidnappers, shipwrecks, sex, marriage, separation, wars, and many other terrifying things are met with resolve, witty comments, and faith that the hero will come, and more often than not, that the heroine will whack someone over the head with a cast-iron skillet and save herself. Because if you let fear take over, you can't let love take over.

We don't really have to fear pirates these days, but we still fear love, even if we claim to want it. As Bjork sings, "It takes courage to enjoy it." I think she's singing about sex, but whether it's love, or reading a romance novel in public or at all . . . it takes courage to conquer fear, or endure ridicule, or even just to let go of whatever might be holding us back. I, for one, cannot imagine going back to a life without love and romance novels.

DO IT: MAKE A LIST OF YOUR FEARS
AND TACKLE ONE OF THEM

What are your worst fears? Heights? Spiders? Public speaking? Flying? Getting cancer? Going somewhere by yourself?

Make a list, write them down and then pick one to focus on. You don't have to pick the hardest one. In fact, it's OK to keep some of your fears safe and sound where they belong. This is not the time to tackle a fear of walking down dark streets alone or getting lost in the desert. Pick something that you know is truly not dangerous, like trying a new hobby. Going someplace new. Saying something you have always wanted to say.

Research your fear a little bit. Why do you think you are afraid of it? Where does your fear come from? A prior bad experience? Something your parents said or did to you? A past-life trauma? If you need help figuring things out, there are some great books on overcoming your fears: *Fearless Living* by Rhonda Britten, who overcame terrible tragedy and fear in her own life, and *Feel the Fear and Do It Anyway*, by Susan Jeffers, Ph.D., who lays out an easy-to-follow plan with *five truths about fear* that we want to share with you here:

1. The fear will never go away as long as I continue to grow.

2. The only way to get rid of the fear of doing something is to go out . . . and do it.

3. The only way to feel better about myself is to go out . . . and do it.

4. Not only am I going to experience fear whenever I'm on unfamiliar territory, but so is everyone else.

5. Pushing through fear is less frightening than living with the underlying fear that comes from a feeling of helplessness.

Of all things to fear, don't be afraid to get and accept help. If you need a friend to go with you, that's OK. If you want to go into therapy to explore this fear, good for you!

But as Susan Jeffers says, the only cure is to do it! Try it. Don't worry, it will all work out just fine and you may just have a fabulous adventure.

LIST: THINGS WE THANKFULLY DON'T HAVE TO BE AFRAID OF ANYMORE, IN THE UNITED STATES, ANYWAY

(Note to reader: The very sad thing is that while most women in developed countries don't have to be afraid of these things anymore, there are still millions of women around the world who do. And it's not money that is stopping change in these issues as much as it's political and religious oppression and lack of education.)

Dying in childbirth. Medea, the heroine of the ancient Greek play of the same name, once declared that she would rather stand in the battle line three times than bear one child. It's a dangerous and deadly event. "During World War I, the number of women who died from the effects of childbirth was greater than the number of men who died on the battlefield" (Gail Collins, *America's Women*). Where is their statue?

Many fatal diseases. Up until the mid 1900s, children in America commonly died from many fatal epidemic diseases like the plague, cholera, typhoid, smallpox, and polio. Yes, AIDS is still rampant in many countries, which also still have these diseases. But affordable treatments are available and these diseases are no longer a guaranteed death sentence.

Losing our children to divorce. It's only in the last hundred years that divorce has become socially acceptable. During the earliest divorces, a woman was not allowed custody of her children (even if the husband was abusive). In the 1800s not only was a woman not allowed to own property, children were considered property and belonged to the husband.

Remaining ignorant. Education for girls and women is a very recent phenomenon. A hundred years ago, vitriolic diatribes were written by men appalled to think that women were even capable of learning. Women weren't allowed to go to college until the 1800s.

Being *legally* beaten and murdered by our husbands or parents. Comparing the lives of fictitious women compared to the real ones she knew, Virginia Woolf writes, "in fact . . . she [the real women of her day] was locked up, beaten and flung about the room." It may not be lawful in some parts of the world, but in others it's common. The World Health Organization cites violence against women as a major health and human rights concern. The phrase "the rule of thumb" came from the days when men were allowed to beat their wife and child with anything narrower than a thumb.

Wearing pants. Joan of Arc was burned at the stake by her own countrymen for wearing pants, and women were not allowed to wear pants in the United States until the early 1900s. Even then it was frowned on. In fact, Jackie Onassis, who always dressed with impeccable style, was once told she couldn't dine in a posh New York City restaurant because she was wearing a pantsuit.

Being forced into marriage. The idea that a person should be allowed to marry for love is so recent and radical that we have yet to comprehend its full impact. In the 1800s feminist Victoria Woodhull spent years in jail for saying women should have the right to mary for love. Throughout the millennia and still today in many countries, women are considered a commodity to be traded for livestock, property, money or status, with no choice and no voice.

Having to work as a prostitute to support yourself. Women were not allowed to "work" until the last hundred years or so, and if for some reason they became destitute because they were orphaned, widowed, or abandoned, often the only means they had of putting food in their mouth and clothes on their back and to support their children was to become a prostitute.

Being ostracized or put to death for having a child out of wedlock. We are especially thankful for this one. It used to happen all the time and, in other countries, still does. A woman in Nigeria who became pregnant after her husband had died recently received international attention because she was slated to be stoned to death.

Not having a vote. It was over a hundred years after the first suffragettes died that women finally got the vote in the United States (1920). In Canada they didn't get it until the 1940s. In many countries, women still don't have it. Even though we have it, many women don't exercise their right.

IN HER OWN VOICE—NANCY DREW

"Unable to speak and hardly able to move, Nancy and Ned could not express their anger aloud. But both were extremely annoyed at themselves for having been captured."

THE SECRET OF THE GOLDEN PAVILION

"The young detective felt a glow of pleasure as always when she made lasting friends of people she had helped."

THE CLUE IN THE DIARY

"I don't align her [Nancy Drew] with the feminist movement at all. That was never in my mind. She was an individual, from start to finish. She was never a person to promote any kind of movement. She was just a person who believed in her own freedom."

THE ORIGINAL CAROLYN KEENE, MILDRED A. WIRT BENSON

PLEASURE REVOLUTIONARY: NANCY DREW, GIRL DETECTIVE

Yes, Nancy Drew is fictional. But she is fearless. For many women she was the first look, the first taste that living successfully and fearlessly was an option. Generations of girls have devoured her books like candy, all two hundred million in print, each time convinced that solving any mystery was not only possible, but exciting and fun.

Nancy Drew was born in a time (the first books debuted in 1930) when many cultural barriers to women had fallen, but few women were claiming new roles. The author of the first few books in the series, and the first to assume the pen name Carolyn Keene, Mildred Wirt Benson said of the character: "She was ahead of her time. She was not typical. She was what the girls were ready for and were aspiring for, but had not achieved." She claimed it and gave the rest of us girls a model to follow. If she could do it, we could at least do some of it.

Nancy did terribly dangerous things—going into strange suspects' homes alone, going scuba diving alone, getting kidnapped, tied up, and gagged in sinking boats. But because of her determination, her ability to stay calm under pressure, and her intelligence, she always got out alive, solved the mystery, and received a hero's salutation. Plus, she wore pretty dresses, drove a cool car, and had lots of friends. Part of Nancy's longevity as a popular character is due to her gender unspecific behavior. She can fix a car in a skirt, accessorized with her level-headed spunk.

We don't think it's a coincidence that Nancy Drew didn't have a mother. Often it's our very own mums who have the strongest influence over us and limit what we think we can do—sometimes even more so than men or culture. Hanna Gruen, the "housekeeper," provided just the right dose of fretful worrying, without any of the authority to demand Nancy stay home. And Nancy's often-absent father gave her the freedom she needed to solve the crime.

The concept of Nancy Drew was created by Edward Stratemeyer, the father of other serial novels like the Hardy Boys. The books he created under the Stratemeyer Syndicate, geared for young readers, fell somewhere between the cheap paperbacks and the overtly moral hard covers. Although they were wildly successful with the kids, librarians often disapproved of them, assuming that they distracted the children from books with more educational value. For a while, Nancy Drew books were banned from public libraries, but eventually they went on to outperform all of Stratemeyer's other series.

The story content and Nancy Drew's personality were created by Mildred Wirt Benson—herself an adventurous character. She was the first woman to attend the University of Iowa and graduated with a masters degree in journalism in 1927. She only wrote twenty-three of the over 350 mysteries published (and solved), and worked as a journalist up until her death. Though many authors have assumed the name of Carolyn Keene, Mildred was the first, and creator of the original girl that millions of readers fell in love with.

Another person to assume the pen name was Harriet Stratemeyer Adams, daughter of Edward. She wrote many more Nancy Drew novels, but also had ghostwriters revise some of the originals to get rid of racial stereotypes, and change Nancy's age from sixteen to eighteen in order to conform to the new driving laws. Nancy's character has also changed bit by bit. Mildred Wirt Benson saw her become more of a "traditional sort of heroine. More of a house type."

Nancy had been created and changed and revised by many authors and a few different publishing companies, but her essence has remained unchanged. She still comes alive with courage *and* femininity, fearlessness *and* friendliness, intelligence *and* common sense. Each book is a page-turner with a not-so-obvious ending. Each, while entertaining, is also a positive encouragement and role model to the little detective in all of us. She knows the secret of the universe—that life is a mystery . . . and we are all detectives.

CHAPTER 3

Be Curious

Pleasure appears when you search for it

TELL ME WHY—MARIA

I think I got stuck in the "why" phase of development. That's the age around two or three years, when kids incessantly ask, "Why?" You can't give them enough answers and you suspect they are doing it just to annoy the heck out of you. Finally, you just have to say, "Because I said so," even though that answer drove you crazy in your own childhood.

But asking why—and not resting till I have the answer—has served me well in life.

My big "why's" started with math. Once math got a bit difficult for me I kept asking the teachers "why do I have to learn this?" The usual answer was "in order to graduate." Not good enough. When I asked my mother she would say "I don't know, I was terrible at math so you probably are too." Basically giving me carte blanche to be a math illiterate. It took tutoring to get me to pass high school math requirements (I passed with a B). But it took an amateur interest in science and a taste of business to finally give me the answers I was looking for.

I'll start with the business side. Yes, I always wanted to be a writer.

But I was also born into a family business. I felt an obligation to learn the business in order to carry on the mission of our family. It was somewhere late at night at the office, my fingers flying across the keyboard while creating a Chopin masterpiece of a spreadsheet, that I had my first mathematical realization: numbers are about relationships. They help you understand how things are in relation to one another. Are people buying more than before or less than before? Why? Do people want what I am selling or don't they? Why? Numbers are a great way of seeing the big picture of relationships . . . but still they don't always tell you why.

Conquering my fear of math enabled me to succeed at my job and be promoted to a job where I worked for both the book and magazine "divisions." And boy, oh boy were they divided. They were constantly fighting with each other and undermining each other. As one of the family owners, I took a step back and looked at the potential long term effect of this division. I realized that our customers were bothered by the inconsistency of our brand between our books and magazines. *Prevention* magazine might say one thing, but a Prevention book something completely different. Or they might both be fighting over that same customer at the same time of year—competing among each other rather than cooperating. So I came up with an idea of organizing our company by brand—for the customer's sake—rather than by media, which made it easier for managers. The response: "You can't do that!"

"Why?"

"Because it's never been done before. If no one else has done it and succeeded what makes you think we can do it?"

If they hadn't been so mean, I probably would have laughed out loud. Instead, I cried. But in retrospect, why should they have listened to me? I was still young (in my thirties). I was the beneficiary of the loathed nepotism. No one *had* done it before, except maybe Martha Stewart—but she only had one brand, we had many (and, as the Guys used to love to say, "She is *such* a bitch"). Plus, I hadn't really run any major business before. In fact, I wasn't even confident that I was right.

But through a long, painful process of coaching, our family decided it was time for a management change, anyway. That change created a domino effect that we were not even sure the company would survive. We hired a new CEO, and consultants were brought in. The new CEO rebuilt a new team of executives, one by one. The team decided that reorganizing by customer group was the right thing to do, and they did a lot of hard work to make it happen—along with a lot of other changes. One of the most important changes was putting the content first. If we created the absolute best products we could, we believed our customers (to whom we were now speaking and marketing in a unified voice) would appreciate it by buying more of our products.

Years later, validation for me came when the *Wall Street Journal* ran a front page story describing Rodale's "unusual operating structure" which our new CEO, Steve Murphy, had restructured "on the basis of the customers they serve rather than their media format." The article, by the way, was about the enormous success of our book *The South Beach Diet*.

I sometimes think that if I hadn't been born into a family business, and I hadn't had a bad start at math, I would have loved to become a scientist. Scientists are always searching for the answers to the question why. It's kind of like a spiritual searching for the meaning of life . . . trying to understand the mystery of it all. But even in science, there is an establishment that doesn't want too many people asking why. And I have come to realize as I talk to scientist friends and the true innovators that I know that after every truly important question of why, there is a ring of fire of ridicule to walk through, a dark tunnel of uncertainty and insults to tread. But on the other side is *the true, deep pleasure of knowing* that there really was a good answer, and you were really right to ask why, and the world (or at least your world) is better off because you did it.

I only wish that when I was little and I asked those math teachers why I needed to learn this, they had said: "Because numbers are the universal language, they are the key to understanding nature and the world, to creating music, and to understanding the relationships of everything to everything else."

Oh yeah, and it also helps you keep track of and manage all the money you make when you succeed (against all odds!) at doing something you truly love.

PANDORA'S "BOX"—MAYA

Once upon a time, there was a naughty demigod named Prometheus. He stole fire from the gods and gave it to humans. Because of Prometheus's thievery, Zeus, the alpha god, decided to punish Prometheus and all men. At the time, women and old age didn't exist in what was considered a golden age. So all the gods and goddesses got together to make Pandora, the first woman, a most beautiful girl. And they gave her all of their own talents and beauty as well as a box filled with the ills of the world. Then they sent her to Prometheus and the men, who had been warned never to accept a gift from the gods. Pandora had been told not to open the box. Naturally the men accepted the present, and Pandora followed her curiosity and opened the box, whereupon all the horrible things that had been packed inside flew out—disease, sadness, suffering, envy, spite—and spread around the world forever altering life as humans had known it. Because of a girl's curiosity and a guy's defiance, the disobedience of a Greek Adam and Eve, the myth implies all of us have to suffer for the rest of eternity. It warns both men and women not to break the rules.

But curiosity has worked out well for me. I can't help but think of all the streets I wandered down, saying, "Oh, what the heck. It looks safe," only to find the best shops, or a fabulous restaurant. And there is nothing like the feeling of turning an unfamiliar corner and coming face to face with a building like the Pantheon, as I did in Rome. That night I also fed my curiosity and tried pistachio gelato for the first time, just because I liked the color. Simply wandering around and remaining open, I found my favorite flavor of ice cream and created one of my happiest memories.

When we're traveling it's easier to be a little more curious. We have on our adventuress hats and anything can happen. But in regular life, acting on curiosity is a little harder, and we invent excuses not to do it. I have invented "research" as an excuse to do anything. The desire to conduct personal research—my curiosity—often overrides my doubts. At times, I've wanted to do something, but wasn't sure it was good to pursue. But then I've said to myself, "Oh, what the heck. I might just get a story out of this." Let's be honest, sometimes it gets me into trouble. But mostly I end up having a great day or a new pair of shoes or a story that will make my friends laugh. You can research yourself into a nap or a life-changing experience.

When I was learning about Pandora in class, everyone kept talking about Pandora's "box." I couldn't help but wonder if box were a metaphor for vagina in ancient Greek as it is in English. I think that the myth of Pandora's box is really about sex. In some versions, she carries a jar instead, like the temple priestesses, which can represent the womb and the sacred power of female sexuality. The box and the girl fascinate men. Yet when men become rabidly curious and act against their better judgment, after they "open" a box—or have sex with a woman or succumb to desire—the myth warns that all the troublesome things in the world will emerge. The male fear of female sexuality and its power has dominated history, and myths had to be invented to illustrate, explain, and justify this fear. Eve and Pandora became the excuse for centuries of subjugation of women.

Why does female sexuality scare men? Perhaps they fear the extreme pleasure we can feel—the clitoris contains some two thousand nerve endings that exist solely for orgasms. If I didn't have one, I would be damn jealous and afraid of it, too. The fear might be even more primal, an awe at women's ability to give birth and our power to create new life, a godlike ability. As far as I know, I have the equipment to give birth, too, but I am still in awe of women who have become mothers. So perhaps men's fear of women's sexual abilities is really the jealousy of a capacity that men can never have.

The Greek myth of Pandora and the Biblical Eve are laced with sexual suggestion—Eve and the serpent, the consciousness she gains of her own nudity, Adam's shame after eating the fruit, his fear of appearing in the nude before God. In this creation myth, Eve's curiosity also feeds the curiosity of men.

It seems as if men created the view that celibacy and virginity are preferable to sex and the fulfillment of pleasure and desire. They make the rules and follow them willingly in order to keep the box closed. Maybe men would have driven themselves crazy wondering what the heck was in that box, but never developing the courage to look or to taste. But women are more subversive. We want to know and we want to feel. We want to be like Eve, taking the bite, and not feeling shame upon the discovery of her nakedness. We want to know whatever

Pandora discovered. And what she discovered, after the horrible things escaped the box, was that hope was also inside. And she let hope out, too, to go flying all over the world, as accessible as any ill.

DO IT: RESEARCH SOMETHING YOU ARE CURIOUS ABOUT

It's truly amazing what you can uncover about life and the world by doing a little bit of research and digging. What's really exciting is when one thing leads to another and you find a whole new understanding of something. Learning and curiosity is a remarkably powerful tool, which is why it's so tightly controlled in cultures where people in power don't want change. Here are five steps to finding something out.

1. *Choose a topic.* Clearly, it should be something you are interested in finding out. Perhaps it's something that has just mystified you since you were a kid.

2. *Do an Amazon.com search.* You will be amazed what does, and doesn't, show up on the screen. Delve into the similar books or customer lists.

3. While you're online, *do a Google search.* Scan through the first few pages of stuff to see if there is anything helpful or good.

4. *Visit your local library or bookstore.* As great as online shopping is, sometimes the serendipity of scanning a book shelf is awesome. You might just find something else you didn't think you were looking for.

5. *Attend a class or workshop to learn more.* Sometimes the best way to understand something is to try it yourself, to talk to experts or other enthusiasts. You'll be happy to know you aren't alone in your curiosity.

All you have to do is ask and the world is open to you. Remember the 5 Ws of reporting: Who, What, Why, Where, and When. Your efforts will take you on an incredible journey.

LIST: THE QUESTIONS WE ASKED OURSELVES
WHICH LED TO US WRITING THIS BOOK

Why is pleasure so often referred to as "guilty pleasures"?

Why are there so many different religions and why do they always fight each other?

Why are romance novels so looked down on by the literary establishment?

Why don't women feel they deserve happy endings?

Who is the black virgin?

Why have women been so suppressed for so long?

Is there a connection between romance novels and the sacred marriage ritual?

Why don't women know more about their history?

When did people begin to fear pleasure and why?

Why is the Virgin Mary the most popular religious figure of all time?

What caused the primal and rabid fear of female sexuality?

Why do we love?

IN HER OWN VOICE: DR. HELEN FISHER

"I came to believe that romantic love is a primary motivation system in the brain—in short, a fundamental human mating drive."

"In one study of middle-aged women, almost 40 percent complained that they were not having enough sex."

"How do you ignite mad romantic passion in another? *Do novel things together.*"

"Romance could not be stifled . . . But the ancient Egyptians, Greeks, Romans, early Christians, Muslims, Indians, Chinese, Japanese, and many others of the historical world usually married for duty, money and alliances, not for love. Indeed, romantic love was feared in much of Asia and parts of Africa. This mercurial force could lead to suicide or homicide; even worse, it could upset the delicate web of social ties."

PLEASURE REVOLUTIONARY: HELEN FISHER, DOCTOR OF LOVE

Love, lust, and romance have fascinated people throughout the ages. Yet "science" usually refused to touch these subjects with a ten-foot pole.

While it seems only natural to want to study love, it took a brave and curious woman to do it: Helen Fisher, a research professor and member of the Center for Human Evolutionary Studies and the anthropology department of Rutgers, has devoted her professional career to understanding why we love. In one of her scientific studies, she scanned the brains of people in love and people who had been dumped, while they were thinking of the other person. She found that love, romance, lust, and sex are not just feelings, but primal human drives, right up there with the need for food, water, and oxygen.

Helen has written four books on the subject: *Why We Love: The Nature and Chemistry of Romantic Love; The First Sex: The Natural Talents of Women and How They Are Changing the World; Anatomy of Love: Natural History of Mating, Marriage, and Why We Stray, Adultery and Divorce;* and *The Sex Contract: The Evolution of Human Behavior.*

We consider her a pleasure revolutionary because her work *is* revolutionary, a result of her asking very simple questions that no other scientist was curious or passionate enough to tackle.

AN INTERVIEW WITH HELEN FISHER

We've heard a lot about the "pleasure center" of the brain. What is it?
Helen: It's called the reward system, and it's basically the dopamine system and all of its networks. But there are probably a lot of other chemicals involved. It's part of the arousal system and strangely enough there are at least five basic brain chemicals associated with reward. For

y to get a reward, you have a very different feeling
a reward. There's a calm and joy in the receiving
v in the getting. But pleasure is basically the
a for winning rewards. You lie in bed at night
urself "How am I going to get him?" *[laughter]*.
tomorrow, what should I wear to school?" You're think-
you're discriminating, you're planning . . . so there's thinking parts
of the reward system for planning and goals. There are emotional re-
gions for feeling joy that he called or despair that he didn't. And then
there are these factories for motivation that keep you saying, "I'm going
to keep trying." *[laughter]*

**We suspect romance novels are addicting. We felt there's got to
be some hormonal reaction and then when we read your book,
we realized it's dopamine! You probably get a buzz of dopamine
every time you read one. They're like potato chips.**
Helen: They're chips in fifty-two countries. *[laughter]* . . . they're
everywhere. It really does do something, there's no question about it.
I'd have to read one to know, which I've never done. If it's the novelty
and the excitement, then it's dopamine.

Are there any harmful, long-term effects of dopamine?
Helen: I would doubt it seriously, but nobody knows. All of the drugs
of abuse drive up dopamine: drinking, cocaine, nicotine, gambling. I
would guess anything that gives you that rush of a high is a dopamine.
Those people don't tend to die of things related to the dopamine system. They tend to die of things related directly to their drug. This
dopamine system, this reward system in the brain is very primitive and
designed to give you that rush regularly so that you go towards the
things you like and away from things you don't like.

It's my guess that dopamine is also associated with creativity. From
the way people behave when they've been rejected [in love]—they're
up all night, they can't sleep, they can't eat, they can't stop thinking—it
really looks like a dopamine high, and a serotonin low. And that's when
you go to your desk in the middle of the night and write poetry.

**You have written that romance and lust are focused so much on
the purpose of reproduction, but in our culture today, as people**

become more educated and affluent it seems we have fewer
children. Why?

Helen: The brain of the rat isn't rushing to reproduce because it believes in evolution and has read *The Origin of Species*. It's doing it because
it feels good. In other words, we have all kinds of conscious motivations,
and we have unconscious payoffs. When it comes to love, the brain is so
deeply patterned to remember, to feel, to hold, because it's so central to
reproduction. So women who fell in love over the millennia tended to
have more children. Those children survived. In other words, something can be selected for simply because it creates more babies. You're
talking about something that is so misunderstood. People don't eat meat
because, a million years ago, eating meat helped their ancestors evolve
bigger brains. They eat meat because it tastes good. But the reason it
tastes good is because there are positive selections for this. People who
liked the taste of meat ended up having more children because meat
helped the metabolism and helped create a bigger brain, and they were
smarter. So it's always a feedback loop. But the long and short of it is,
no, [when] the vast majority of people the vast majority of the time
climb into bed with somebody, the last thing they want is babies. *[laugh-
ter]* But still, liking sex and falling in love, those people end up having
more babies and those babies lived and passed on this taste for sex and
love.

Why do you think the whole idea of pleasure and romance has
been so scorned?

Helen: Because it is so powerful. In hunting and gathering societies,
generally the first marriage is arranged, but it's arranged among very
young people, they generally break up and then kids go on to pick their
partners for themselves. So romance just carries on. And it's not
scorned and sexuality isn't scorned and everybody has their rules of sex.
I think the huge transition is when we settled down on the farm. Because you've got a fixed piece of real estate [and] a huge shift in who
did what on the farm. Men had to move the rocks, fell the trees, pile
the wood, and bring the food off to the local markets and then they
come home with resources—the equivalent of money. And women lost
their ancient ability to wander off and provide 60 to 80 percent of the
evening meal. They were relegated to second-class jobs of picking,
weeding, pruning, and preparing the evening meal. They had to have

lots of babies because suddenly children were essential for work. Women became much less economically independent, with farming. And when you take a look around the world at farming societies, women's status is lower than men's. In the industrial revolution, women started moving back into the job market, and I think we're really returning to the kinds of power relations that we had a million years ago when women would come home with just as much "money." And money is power. You can walk out if you have it, and you cannot walk out if you don't. So long and short, with the beginning of farming, you really do see a shift.

In those societies farming with a hoe, women are extremely powerful, still. Even at the turn of the twentieth century when data was beginning to be collected in Africa women were extremely powerful, they were the farmers. With the beginning of plow agriculture, the farm became men's work. And so men's roles became extremely powerful and women's role became less economically essential, although they were quite essential, but secondary roles.

When you suddenly begin to collect property, then you want to hand your property to your children, and then you want to have the quite important rule of inheritance. And when you start having to have property that needs to be inherited and divided up then you've got to curtail sexuality. And it's more important to curtail female sexuality because if your young boy has extra children by another woman, that's just passing your seed to other women, that's Darwinianly great. But if you stick all your money and time and effort in your wife who is your helpmate, living on what you inherited, and she starts having babies with a different man and you're cuckolded, then your property's not going to go to your own genetic lineage. So you really see in agrarian cultures around the world female sexuality much more curtailed than male sexuality—among those who have money. We're always hearing about those with money.

What do you think the role of religion plays in all this?
Helen: Religion is an absolutely fascinating mechanism for social control. It sets standards, it defines the in-group from the out-group. It ostracizes offenders; it celebrates those who toe the line. Religion does so many things. The most powerful concept the human animal has ever come up with is God. It's much more powerful than the gun, or

Kleenex or the ballpoint pen. The concept of God has done more to unite people and to divide people and look, it still is. And you can commit horrible cruelty and feel good about it. It's the belief in god and the belief that your god is the right god. It's absolutely terrifying. Religion not only keeps the status quo together, but it's a wonderful reflection of people's beliefs. I think we're going to move forward to having more female gods. I don't really trace religion, but there's every reason to think that five hundred years from now, Mary will be more powerful. And then other kinds of females will come in. Because women are becoming more powerful! They're reclaiming their ancient power.

Were you raised in any kind of religion?
Helen: Absolutely. We were part of the Congregational Church. But it didn't stick on Helen Fisher. In the eighth grade, every girl in my class was supposed to take confirmation and I was the only girl who absolutely refused to do it. I just didn't get it. I don't mind if other people do it, as long as they don't plague me with it and plague everybody else with it. *[laughter]* Why is it that that the human animal needs to have everybody else believe the way they do? It's some tribal thing, you're either with us or against us. I don't think I'm going anywhere when I die. It's dust to dust. How wonderful it would be to believe in all that.

So do you practice any religion? How would you describe yourself now?
Helen: Raging atheist. *[laughter]* My boyfriend likes to go to church and I like to go with him. It's something that we do together. I don't mind, I think it's bizarre. I love music and I love pretty flowers and I like people being friendly and all of that. But it is no different from me going into the Episcopal Church around the corner, which I can do, than going to a Navajo peyote ceremony. You know, I don't understand that one anymore than I understand this one on some emotional level. But I can still get tremendous joy out of the going. And crazily enough, I like to pray.

But I don't think prayer has to do with God. The female brain lives easily with ambiguity. And people say, "Well who are you praying to?" and I say, "Oh the forces of the universe." I mean, what difference does it make? When I pray for somebody, I feel better. If I feel better maybe they will feel better.

What are the things that give you the most pleasure?
Helen: I get a lot of pleasure out of a lot of things. I love my daily walk in the park, love seeing the seasons change day by day as I go through that park. I love the sound of the birds. I love taking my hot bath. I love being the right weight. God. *[laughter]* Doesn't happen a lot. And my blue jeans. I love butter. *[laughter]*. I love my steamed broccoli. I just love the foods that I eat. I love to travel with the man that I go out with. I love to look at people. My work is a great deal of fun when it's all over. *[laughter]* I love public transportation, I love to see all the people. These are the simple things in life.

What about your life led you on this path of questioning and seeking answers?
Helen: No one's ever asked me this. Although I had a very turbulent relationship with my mother, she was definitely very curious and interested in a huge number of things. Both my parents were upper-class Connecticut, but very down to earth, regular people. They really liked sex. *[laughter]* I just didn't grow up with feeling that sex was dirty. I've got my own values of right and wrong, but sexuality to me just doesn't ring the American chimes of sin.

I guess the only other thing I would say is that I grew up in this glass house, and everyone else had a glass house and by the time I was six I used to sneak into the woods and sit on the stone wall by myself and watch my neighbors eat dinner. *[laughter]*. It was like my TV. And somebody said to me, "You know, there's a science for people like you." *[laughter]*. Anthropology.

CHAPTER 4

Discover What You Like and Don't Like

Pleasure is personal

THE LONG AND TORTUROUS PROCESS
OF FINDING OUT—MARIA

Actually, I'm amazed at how little my likes and dislikes have changed since I was a kid. Here is what I like: soft blankets, homemade soup, the smell of oil paints and a good portrait, writing, mud, reading, swimming in clear blue water, drinking coffee, animals, music of all kinds, and traveling. Here is what I don't like: being teased, doing laundry, folding grocery bags, mean people, bigotry and prejudice, drunkenness, swimming in dark dirty water, not having coffee.

But let's face it, when most people hear the word pleasure, they think of sex. Yet nothing is more symbolically fraught with mixed emotions. Why do we feel shame and embarrassment? Why do we prefer to grow up in ignorance—avoiding all discussion and learning about it?

My own sexual history is painful to remember. I wasn't abused or violently raped. But growing up with a mother who was absorbed in her own personal journey and who often drank to deal with her frustration, with a distant father, and coming of age at the height of the "sexual revolution" was not a good thing. I always say that the revolution in the 1970s was just that a girl wasn't allowed to say "no." In 1976, at fourteen, I'd already fooled around in boys' basements after school and had no cherry left to pluck, but an adult man who I thought was being friendly took whatever was left that year. I do think of it as a rape. Legally, it was rape. I did not set out that evening to have sex. I had no protection or self-esteem to prevent anything. I don't remember having any talks with my parents, or lessons in school, or advice. It was like I was blindly, ignorantly set free in a world I had no idea how to navigate in.

From there I gave in to a series of misadventures. Back seats of cars and vans. More basements. Strange beds. Through it all, I wondered why I didn't feel anything. I had plenty of desire. In fact I was raging with it. But when it came to the act—I might as well have been watching TV, which, lots of times, I was. I felt no pleasure.

My first real boyfriend was Maya's "bio-dad." While he didn't give me my first orgasm, the first orgasm I had with him came quite by accident long after we were first sexually active. It surprised us both. Eventually he became quite good at it. But that didn't mean I wanted to marry him when I got pregnant. He wanted his freedom and, frankly, I did too. In our relationship I had felt that I had lost my true self, my independence, my spirit. I felt rather lucky that I had been so active for so long and not gotten pregnant sooner.

When I told a relative I was keeping my baby, she told me I would never have another boyfriend again, that no one would want a single mother with a kid. She was wrong.

After Maya was born, I moved on to a series of longer relationships. In one, the sex was technically proficient, but there was no passion. In another, there was so much passion I practically exploded with it, but almost everything else about the relationship was horrible. I had a few more one-night stands just to remind myself how awful they were and then I made a vow. No more sex until I found true love.

I had always believed in true love when I was younger and have never let go of that belief. But at that time I wasn't sure what it meant anymore. So, I spent over two years really working on myself, trying to build some self-esteem, self-love, and respect in order to understand how to make true love. I thought I had found it when I met a guy who I followed to Vermont (still no sex, though), which led me to the insight I needed. He was a handsome, adventurous mountain climber getting his masters degree in Sacred Mountains from Harvard (whatever that meant!). One night, we were sitting and talking in a Vermont meadow beneath a starry, moonlit sky under a maypole (symbol of an ancient goddess fertility festival), when I realized that I had been looking for too much in another person. I was looking for someone to complete me. The real reason I was attracted to him was that I wanted to be him. Or just like him. I realized that I wanted to be complete in myself, first. I had to stop putting my dreams on hold and start living them.

Not much later, I met Lou, my husband. But the point is, I might not have recognized him before that maypole incident. With Lou, I realized that pleasure and love evolve. I evolve. He evolves. True love is when both people have room to grow and evolve together and enjoy the journey (not without its bumps and crying fits, however!). True love is when you find someone with whom you can be your true self.

One of the reasons I am obsessed with historical romances is that they (almost) always have the absolute perfect scene where she loses her virginity to the hero. He pleasures her first, he treasures her, she feels total passion and desire, her orgasm is a religious experience—and so is his.

I mourn my lost virginity and innocence and try to guard it fiercely in my own daughters. And I think wouldn't it be nice if we lived in a world where boys would learn how to give pleasure instead of how to fight and kill. Wouldn't it be lovely if our daughters could expect their first experience to be transforming and joyful—not necessarily within the bounds of marriage, but within the bounds of self-respect and love. Wouldn't it be nice if we didn't expect our children, starting from ignorance, to figure it out by trial and error.

It would be nice. And we can decide to make this happen.

YOU DON'T HAVE TO LIKE IT. JUST TRY IT—MAYA

"You don't have to like it, just try it," was the dinner table refrain in our house. "But Mom," I would say, "I tried it last week and I didn't like it." I was then silenced with the "five more bites" rule. And even though I pretended to hate whatever I was forced to try, and

I pretended to roll my eyes every time that line was uttered, it did have a certain amount of sense and fairness to it.

The other night, my mum and I went out to a Japanese restaurant. Since everything on the menu looked absolutely delicious, yet scary and foreign at the same time, and I was too tired to make a decision, I ordered the tasting menu, figuring, what the hell. Just try anything and everything. See if I like it.

The first course was green beans in sesame sauce, which is a very good combination of taste and texture. There was a cold seafood salad with mostly raw scallops that tasted like salt water. Usually, I don't like scallops, but I ate them anyway, and I did enjoy them. I ate some squid—my favorite pieces are the ones with violet colored tentacles simply because they are kind of scary. Somehow, scary foods taste a little bit better and stronger than familiar foods. Perhaps it's the attitude that goes with trying them that is so satisfying. Sea urchin came out next. One of the scariest foods with its bright orange color, and a consistency like partially melted Jell-O—you have to grab a bit of it with your chopsticks, wiggle it around, and then slurp it up and let the taste of the ocean wash over your mouth. I felt very adventurous, and imagined that all the other diners are in awe of my daring.

The final course was cold soba noodles made from organic buckwheat hand-ground right on the premises, with a special dipping sauce. I think that I will never have better soba in my entire life, but lord knows I'll try just to see.

Yes, it is only dinner. But it is a safe, rewarding way to test my Mom's mantra, "You don't have to like it, just try it." That way, if you don't like it, you know you made an effort, and can walk away without guilt. I have also tried to apply this philosophy to other aspects of my life—like colleges, boys, books, movies, and furniture set-ups. You might affirm that, yes that boy is definitely a toad and not a prince, but you also might discover something new and wonderful.

DO IT: MAKE A LIST OF EVERYTHING YOU REALLY LIKE AND REALLY DON'T LIKE

We women are taught that we are not supposed to hate anything, but in truth there are things we like and don't like, and they interfere with pleasure. Actually, we women are taught that we are supposed *not* to hate certain things—cooking, obedience, being nice, and home decorating. Then we are taught that we are supposed to hate other things—mainly hot and dirty sex, and the men who can provide it. Now is your chance to wipe the slate clean and make your own list.

Take out a piece of paper. Write "love it" on one side and "hate it" on another. Draw a line down the middle and start writing. Don't censor yourself. Realize that if you put something on the hate side of the list you will not be struck down with lightning and be sent directly to hell. Let yourself go. Nothing is too big or too small. Be specific. Do you really hate your sister or do you just hate it when she blames you for everything? Don't make a value judgment, just let go and see what you discover about yourself.

Here's the fun part: If there are things on the "hate it" list that you can stop doing—stop doing what you don't like! If you hate doing laundry, send it out. If you hate cleaning the toilet, hire a cleaning lady or get your kids or husband to do it. If you hate your job, find a new one. If you hate your family, stop hanging out with them.

Keep your list handy and add to it when you think of something. Examine it every once in a while. Sometimes, just the act of recording it can free you. Sometimes, the things you hate become the things you love, once you try them or start to understand it. Sometimes you just still hate them. That's OK.

LIST: TEN THINGS WORTH TRYING

Sushi. You don't have to eat the stuff with the raw fish in it. Try avocado roll, with a bit of soy sauce, ginger, and wasabi. It's delish.

Tofu. Prepared properly, it's completely edible and in fact, really, good. We suggest fried tofu with some salt and spices of your choice.

Brussels sprouts. Again, preparation is everything. We've gotten teenage boys to love them. Boil for three minutes. Cut in half. Saute in butter, olive oil and garlic. Sprinkle with romano cheese and bread crumbs. Salt. Yum.

Horseback riding. How you relate to a horse is how you relate to your life. If you are terrified and avoid horses completely it's worth looking at what else you are avoiding in your life. If you can conquer your fear and get on and ride . . . well, the world is your oyster.

Country music. Country gets the same bad rap among the social and literary elite that romance novels do. The stereotype is that it's for hicks, Republicans, and fundamentalist Christians. It's actually quite good. A great way to sample it is XM Satellite Radio, Channel 11, the Nashville station. With satellite radio, if you hear a song you like you can see who it is right away. Start with Kenny Chesney, Martina McBride, and Keith Urban.

Romance novels. Speaking of romance novels . . . not all of them are great, but a lot of them are. If you are just starting out, try Julia Quinn. She's our favorite.

A different faith's religious service. Get outside your own box. You will not be struck down by lightning and you may actually learn something. If your own faith can't stand up to the exposure to other religions and to comparison with them, then maybe it's not right for you. You may need to ask yourself some questions about what you want from your religious practice.

Massage. You can get all different kinds these days (just don't call the numbers from a highway billboard). Lots of doctors even recommend therapeutic massage to help with healing and pain management. Try a hot stone massage, where smooth warm stones rest on your body. Or if you are feeling adventurous, a cranial-sacral massage, which focuses on your skull and scalp, can often dislodge old memories.

Sex outdoors. Ah, the breeze on your naked skin, the warm sun on your body, the thrill of possibly getting caught . . . having sex outside is a reminder that we are partaking in an ancient, primal act shared by almost every living species. In fact, there are probably some birds and bees doing it right next to you. It's an orgy!

Internet porn. Speaking of orgies, the Internet is a treasure trove of them. Women tend to have a knee-jerk negative reaction to the idea of porn, but the fact is more and more sites about sex are created by women, for women, and catering to women's unique needs, fantasies, and interests. Before you form an opinion about Internet porn, it's worth checking it out yourself. (See chapter 20 for our suggestions.)

Then, at least, you can form an educated opinion. Plus, it's a fascinating place to explore and discover just how normal you really are. Clearly, if you have kids using the same computer as you do, put parental controls on it. But then, since you are the parent, you can sneak around them.

IN HER OWN VOICE: VERONICA FRANCO

"Since true love consists above all in the union of a lover's soul and will with those of the beloved, and since the commitment of feigned love cannot lay claim to the correspondence of true love, I advise you to profit from my telling you the truth, for this, too, is a mark of affection."

"When we too are armed and trained, we can convince men that we have hands, feet, and a heart like yours; and although we may be delicate and soft, some men who are delicate are also strong; and others, coarse and harsh, are cowards. Women have not yet realized this, for if they should decide to do so, they would be able to fight you until death; and to prove that I speak the truth, amongst so many women, I will be the first to act, setting an example for them to follow; and on you who have sinned against them all, I turn with whichever weapon you may choose, with the wish and hope of throwing you to the ground."

"I transform my mad love into friendship, and thinking of your immense gifts, I reshape my soul to emulate you; and if my thoughts on this were known to you, you would not let my honest and temperate desires go unfulfilled."

PLEASURE REVOLUTIONARY: VERONICA FRANCO— THE SACRED PROSTITUTE

It's been called the world's oldest profession. Back in ancient times, prostitutes were much like priests—for a small donation, they offered salvation, confession, forgiveness, and a moment of peace. In fact, they were called priestesses. In the first hero's journey, the five-thousand-year-old *Epic of Gilgamesh*, a wild man is civilized by making love to a sacred prostitute who is sent by the king. Since ancient times, billions and billions of women—some sacred prostitutes, street prostitutes, courtesans, wives, mistresses, and girlfriends—have attempted the same feat of "civilizing" their men. As the romance author Nicole Jordan writes in the *Romantic Times Bookclub* magazine, "It's the primal romance fantasy for many women—taking on the challenge of civilizing the savage beast in a man and teaching him to value love." Apparently we still have work to do.

As times changed, and religion became more patriarchal, the sacred prostitutes were kicked out of the temples. But because proper women were expected to be nonsexual except to conceive children, the demand for prostitution grew. For many women who could not afford a dowry for marriage (in most cultures a woman's family had to pay a man to marry her) the only option available to support herself was prostitution.

The world of prostitution has a hierarchy, at the top of which are mistresses and courtesans who offer beauty, intelligence, and a level of passion and companionship many good, proper ladies were not thought able or accustomed to provide. Venice in the 1500s was renowned for its courtesans, and Veronica Franco was the most venerated. Veronica Franco is our representative of all the prostitutes, from the sacred to the profane, a shining jewel in the long chain of women who used their beauty, intelligence, and sexuality to survive.

Veronica Franco was a rare woman in the Renaissance world of men who was able to carve out a literary and historic place for herself. In an oppressive environment for all women—there were laws regulating the clothes and jewelry they wore, and married women were prohibited from speaking in public—Veronica Franco, literary courtesan, emerged.

The social position of a courtesan at this time would seem odd to us today. Courtesans were not mere prostitutes, trading money for sex. They were the most highly educated women, and often charged a fee simply for conversation. Their sumptuous dress often resembled the outfits of noble women, creating some confusion on the streets. They, like male courtiers of the time, depended on the patronage of wealthy individuals to live and pursue their art. And so, it was the male courtiers who most condemned the courtesans, who had a key advantage in the competition for patronage—sex.

Veronica was born to a professional family, and her mother had been a courtesan. She had three brothers, and it is assumed that she was able to share in their education. After a bad arranged marriage to a doctor, Veronica entered into the life of a courtesan (with her mother's encouragement).

In the 1570s Veronica became involved with Domenico Venier, who presided over a renowned literary salon, which she often hosted in her own home. In 1575 she published a volume of poetry, *Terze Rime*, in which seventeen of twenty-five poems are hers. In 1580 she published a volume of personal letters, in which she commented on public life, on the situation and position of women in her time, and reflected on her own experiences. She published her thank-you letter to the great painter Tintoretto for his portrait of her, and wrote to Henry III, King of France, who was reputed to be one of her lovers and to have chosen her above all others to spend time with while in Venice. Perhaps 10 percent of the female population of Renaissance Venice was literate, so their writings might have had a limited audience. Yet Veronica's writings were exchanged and discussed in the salons by the most important male thinkers, artists, and writers of her day. She always supported women, and used her platform as a writer to speak out for them, often reaching an audience other women never could.

Shortly after she survived trumped-up charges that cost her her fortune, she died at the age of forty-five. Her will, drafted at the age of twenty-four, made generous provisions for her family, as well as the women of Venice with limited means and opportunities.

Some writers and historians have romanticized the life of the courtesan and mistress, which was almost always difficult. Veronica's own description, written to a mother considering putting her daughter into the profession, was this: "It is a most wretched thing, contrary to human reason, to subject one's body and industriousness to a servitude whose very thought is most frightful. To become the prey of so many, at the risk of being despoiled, robbed, killed, deprived in a single day of all that one has acquired from so many over such a long time, exposed to many other dangers of receiving injuries and dreadful contagious diseases; to eat with another's mouth, sleep with another's eyes, move according to another's will, obviously rushing toward the shipwreck of one's mental abilities and one's life and body; What greater misery? What riches, what comforts, what delights can possibly outweigh all this? Believe me, of all the world's misfortunes, this is the worst."

But at the end of her life, exiled to the country estate of one of her lovers, she was unrepentant. According to Betsy Prioleau in her book, *Seductress*, Veronica " imagines an erotic earthly paradise where lascivious murals decorate the walls, desire and friendship merge, and the sexes live in equality and sensuous harmony. In such a utopia the courtesan redeems society with the 'positive power of her love.'" At this time, it was almost impossible even for a courtesan to imagine a day when sexual pleasure and love could be shared without the exchange of property and money. In fact, it would take more than another four hundred years.

CHAPTER 5

Examine Your Religion

Pleasure is embedded in the roots of all religions, but threatened in the translation

> *If women are ordained, clericalism will return. There is no love in the [women's ordination] movement, only a thirst for power.*
> —A PRIEST IN HIS THIRTIES FROM
> THE SCRANTON, PENNSYLVANIA, DIOCESE, *ALLENTOWN*
> *MORNING CALL*, OCTOBER 21, 2000

LOSING MY RELIGION, FINDING MY FAITH—MARIA

I remember the exact moment I decided I could no longer be a Lutheran. I was sitting in church, doodling pictures of Jesus on my church program, as usual, when it sunk in just what the minister was saying. He was trashing women. While I don't remember his exact words, the gist of it was that a woman should be obedient and submissive to her husband. That all women, like Eve, the original bad girl, were the cause of all suffering. I thought to myself, how can he possibly be saying these things about women in 1975!

Even my mother was furious enough after that sermon to quit the church, and she had been the most popular Sunday School teacher for adults. In fact, maybe the minister was aiming his little chat at her, now that I think about it. We never went back.

main message was that we should love each other and that God loves us. As I continued my research on different religions and their history, I felt like a detective trying to solve a mystery while missing the biggest clue.

The violence upset me the most. Why did the Church wage so many bloody wars? "Heretics" were throughout the church's history thrown to the lions, burned at the stake, tortured, and murdered. Hundreds of Protestants had their heads chopped off because they believed an individual had the right to read the Bible in their own language. Women in all religions were being sold, traded, raped, murdered (legally), stoned, and forced into bigamous marriages all while being blamed for all the sins of the world.

Many good things have come out of religion, and many good, faithful people embodied and acted on the best of the beliefs. But I was still looking for some bigger answers and reasons. I was still asking, why? Although I hadn't completely lost my faith, I just didn't know what to believe in. I was depressed and disgusted.

Then Lou, Maya, Eve, and I traveled to Japan. The first day, a tour guide took us around Tokyo. We kept passing little shrines on street corners and temples tucked between office buildings. It was the first time ever that I (and my family) were the only Caucasians we saw.

The guide told us that "Japanese are Buddhist on the day they are born and the day they die, but the rest of their lives they are Shinto." Never heard of it. The Japanese culture was so different. My husband found a Catholic church in Kyoto to go to, and I was struck by the similarity of that church and service to the ones in the United States, same words, same props, same smell. There, I realized any religion that believes its way is the right way is like a brand trying to increase its market share in each new country. The contrast between the sameness of that church service, and the total differentness right outside the church door was startling. I wasn't sure what to make of it, but it didn't make me feel good.

Later, however, on Miyajima, a little island in southern Japan, I found my faith again. We were climbing Mount Misen to see two incredible sites, a temple that had kept a fire burning for over a thousand years and a monkey preserve. On the ground, at every turn, and in every special place we came upon little shrines with coins, candles, and even kewpie dolls. The mountain seemed alive with all the love

After that Sunday, I took a little sabbatical from religion for ab(
a year. It was a nice break from the Sunday morning obligation. Bu
also started to question things. Why did that minister feel it was ok
to trash women? Why were women being blamed for all the sins of th
world? What did we do that was so terrible to deserve the wrath of th
church? Were other religions more appreciative of women and bette.
for us? The really big question for me was, is there something, a universal truth, common to all religions?

I began, over twenty years ago, to search for answers. And, this
search is still going strong. I read books on Jesus' life. I read religious
history books. I took classes in college. I delved into Cabala and
Sufism. I studied astrology and the mystics. I read the Bible and the
Other Bible, which includes all the sacred and historical texts that
were edited out of the Bible. I visited cathedrals, temples, and sacred
sites around the world. I went to the Vatican and the Pantheon,
Notre Dame in Paris and my grandfather's temple on the Lower East
Side. I slept in a kiva on the Ute reservation in Colorado. I read *The
Religions of the World* by Huston Smith, a great expert on world religions, and took a course with him at the Omega Institute. I studied
Iyengar yoga for five years. I tried vegetarianism for a few years. I
even was celibate for two years. I looked into Buddhism. Being one-
quarter Jewish, I thought maybe I really was supposed to continue on
that path so I looked into that. My grandmother was a French
Huguenot, so I studied their interesting history, which is the story of
the persecution of Protestants by the Catholics. When I met my husband, who was raised to be a devout Roman Catholic, I attended some
of his ceremonies (including a required marriage preparation course),
but because of what I had learned studying the French Huguenots I
found it hard to support Catholicism. I studied the history of the
Moravians, who started our daughter's school over 250 years ago,
serious Protestants who have a "Love Feast" ceremony, which, I have
to say, is one of my favorites (coffee and cake in church!).

After almost two decades of searching, I still had no answers to
some fundamental questions: Why do the major religions denigrate
women, and treat sex and almost anything pleasurable with suspicion
and condemnation? And why are all the histories of religions filled
with such bloody, vengeful, horrible violence? As I discovered, even
love is not a common theme in these histories, even though Jesus'

and appreciation that people had for it and had expressed and made visible over thousands of years. I couldn't believe that a place and a people could be so very different from everything I had known before, so vital, so magical.

I didn't convert to Shinto, but I realized that the Being I believed in had made *everything* and *everyone:* Shinto and Catholic, Jew and Palestinian, love and hate, Muslim and Hindu, creation and revolution, Japanese and Americans. . . . I didn't have a name for my faith, but I also didn't need one.

A few years later, when I read the Old Testament, I was surprised to discover over and over that the Shinto practices seemed much like the ones that the Jews had been trying to destroy: worshiping under every tree, at every high place, burning incense. It made me realize how much we have yet to discover about our true history.

I still didn't have all the answers. But I had faith that I would find them.

WHAT'S SO FUNNY ABOUT PEACE, LOVE, AND UNDERSTANDING?—MAYA

G grew up without a church but I did not grow up without spirituality, faith, hope, or love. And that, I think, made all the difference.

I was exposed to many forms of "official" worship: Lutheran and Catholic services, Moravian Love Feasts (food in church!), my great-grandmother's Jewish funeral, my sister's Catholic baptism. A class in high school that examined all the world's religions took us on field trips to a Buddhist temple in Pennsylvania where we meditated and later to Muslim prayer services. In the parking lot before entering the mosque all of us girls helped each other arrange our head scarves. I chanted in Sanskrit at yoga classes and noticed the statues and art in my Hindu friends' homes.

In spite of these experiences as a teenager, I mostly learned about religion rationally and logically, from books about the people of various religions and the history of the Catholic Church's revised beliefs and Martin Luther's scandalous idea that an individual could get to God without an intermediary. I read the Bible and books about the Bible. I saw the hurt and the pain and restriction and martyrdom and rules that made no sense. (But then again, I was a teenager and thought most everything was stupid.) These major religions seemed to me to exalt renunciation and feeling bad, and although I did feel frustrated, unhappy, and dissatisfied with my life, I didn't think renouncing the world was going to make me feel better. I was asking, along with Elvis Costello, "What's so funny about peace, love, and understanding?" because, frankly, for all the talk of God's love, I wasn't getting it. The religions made God just seem like an asshole with arbitrary rules and demands to renounce the things that did make me happy.

But I still had a belief in something fabulous and magical, so I decided to read books that presented a different picture from that of the traditional histories. I read novels. I read books about Mary and ancient goddess worship, because my mom kept leaving them around the house. And in those books I found a religion that seemed way cooler than all the boy religions: goddess worship. Because goddess worship was so ancient and largely unstudied, the rules weren't as clear, but they did involve sex and worship, and belief in the power of creativity. Like Mother Mary, the goddesses were mothers who gave you a metaphysical hug when you felt sad or bad. So, when no one was looking, I started talking and praying to Mary and believing in the power of girls.

When I turned twenty-one, my dad sent me a special birthday letter to accompany his gift, a collection of beautiful leather-bound, gold-embossed sacred texts: the Bible, the Koran . . . all of 'em. This is what he wrote in the accompanying letter: "Just one warning, don't look for faith in a book (not even one bound in leather with gold embossing). It's not there. It's a gift you have to ask for—and one you have to be wise enough to accept when it is offered." He goes to Mass every Sunday. He's devout, but not holier than thou. And he's right. I didn't find my faith until I stopped looking for it in books and started praying when I felt like it. And with each prayer, I felt a little better and believed a little more.

One night, faith, hope, and love came through for me: It was a Saturday night and I was at work. The offices were on the eighth floor of an office building, empty except for me and a co-worker, who happened to be my boyfriend. I decided to take my break and wander around the floor. In back, there is a sort of enclosed fire escape, with a door that locks behind you, so it had to be propped open. There was also a door to another stairwell, that, if opened, set off an alarm. Often I would go out there on my break because it was quiet and had a nice view of the city. But that night, I forgot to prop open the door, and I got locked in. I opened the door to the stairs figuring I would just leave the building in back and come in through the front door. The alarm went off, and I ran down eight flights of stairs only to find a locked metal door that even God couldn't break through. So I ran back upstairs (in three-inch heels, mind you) trying every door on every floor. They were all locked. I got back up to my little fire escape (I had remembered to prop that door open, thank god). For a moment I debated crying, but then reasoned that wouldn't help. I did, however, panic that I would end up in the "Weird But True" section of the newspaper, which would have been worse than being locked in a fire escape for days.

There were only two things left for me to do: pray to Mary and pound on the door. I prayed for Mary to give my boyfriend/co-worker a bad feeling, and to come looking for me. When he came out into the hall, he would hear my banging on the door, and follow his curiosity. And after forty-five minutes of nonstop pounding on the door, he pushed it open and I fell into his arms. He said he was glad I was OK, because he had a bad feeling in his stomach . . . he said all this before I had even told him I had prayed to Mary for the exact thing. I gave him a kiss, and sent up a thank-you prayer to Mary.

I finally learned the power of faith, love, and prayer by getting rescued from a locked fire escape.

DO IT: PRETEND YOU HAD TO CREATE
YOUR OWN RELIGION

Imagine for a moment that you were raised without any idea of the religion you know today. Imagine for a moment that nothing terrible would happen if you invented your own religion . . . in fact, you would be especially blessed. Imagine there was no sin (of course, if you wanted to you could create it as part of your religion), no concept of heaven and hell, no ancient traditions you were trained to fulfill.

How would you feel? Lost in the wilderness? Free at last?

Here are some questions to ask your self. You may want to come back to this page at the end of our book and see if you would change things a bit.

1. What are the most important values or virtues in your religion?

2. Are there practices you would do every day?

3. Are there weekly, monthly, or seasonal things you would celebrate?

4. Is your religion one that you would practice alone or with other people?

5. Does your religion have any sins? If so, what are they?

6. What is most sacred to you?

7. Is there an afterlife or reincarnation in your beliefs?

8. What role does nature play in your religion?

9. How would you treat men and women differently, or would you?

10. How would your religion be most different from all the others?

LIST: SIX THINGS RELIGION GOT RIGHT

While there are many things in the history of religions that were not as stellar as we would like them to be, there are a few things that religion has gotten right.

Love. Many religions do put love in the forefront, where it belongs. Loving god, loving your neighbor, and loving yourself—it's hard to go wrong with love.

Charity. The idea of serving others and helping each other is not only important, but it's a pleasure. When you really help someone who needs it, you feel good.

Tolerance. When it works, it's magic, and it's what makes America so great. All of us, Jews, Catholics, Muslims, Italians, Irish, pagans, and all the rest, live in peace and harmony side by side.

Forgiveness. And its sister, compassion, are blessings when they are achieved. Forgiving others, and yourself, and feeling forgiven is one of the best, most pleasurable feelings there is. Spread it around.

Prayer. Studies have shown that even if you don't believe in a god, praying—even for people you have never met—does really work. Maybe it's the power of sending your energy out into the universe, but it's good for you and the world.

Singing. The wonder of a place of worship filled with a chorus of song is truly one of the most spiritual moments of life. It doesn't have to be in a church, either.

IN HER OWN VOICE: RIANE EISLER

"Candles, music, flowers, and wine—these we all know are the stuff of romance, of sex and of love. But candles, flowers, music, and wine are also the stuff of religious ritual, of our most sacred rites. . . . Is it just accidental that *passion* is the word we use for both sexual and mystical experiences? Or is there here some long-forgotten but still powerful connection?"

"Changes in consciousness are a very strange thing. Suddenly we see what has been there all the time. And we wonder how it could for so long have been invisible to us."

"The critical factors in politically repressive societies are, first, the repression of female sexual freedom and, second, the distortion of both male and female sexuality through the erotization of domination and violence."

"To heal ourselves, we also have to heal society."

"For our ancestors, both life and pleasure were within the realm of the sacred. In short, I believe that . . . our ancestors sacralized pleasure, particularly that most intense physical pleasure we are given to feel: the pleasure of sexual ecstasy."

PLEASURE REVOLUTIONARY: RIANE EISLER,
PROFESSOR OF PLEASURE

Without Riane Eisler, we could not have written or even conceived of this book.

A prominent cultural historian and evolutionary theorist, Eisler has written numerous books, including *The Chalice and the Blade* and *Sacred Pleasure*, and analyzed women's global history. Looking closely at ancient artwork, artifacts, religions, and the world around her, Eisler discovered the power of women and pleasure, examined how we as a culture have forgotten that link between women and pleasure, and why we need to rediscover it. She has also put forth a new model of growth and governance for our culture—partnership, rather than dominance, in every relationship: man/woman; husband/wife; parent/child; community/state; nation to nation.

Born in Vienna, Riane fled to Cuba with her parents to escape the Nazis. She eventually emigrated to the United States, where she earned degrees in law and sociology from the University of California, taught at the University of California, serves on numerous boards, and has done pioneering work in human rights.

AN INTERVIEW WITH RIANE EISLER

How did you come to write *Sacred Pleasure*?
Riane: I had this insight that if you analyze all of the various ways that we classify how we live and what societies we live in, they're either held together by pleasure, by neutral gods, by sharing, caring, and joy, or they're held together by these rankings of control, of domination, which are ultimately motivated by the fear of pain. So then I really got into the idea of pain versus pleasure. There will always be pain. But I'm talking about a revolution of a way of living, a social system, belief systems, [to get away from] institutions that keep perpetuating the infliction and the suffering of pain.

How do you define power in the dominator or partnership model of society?
Riane: There are two ways of looking at power. There is certainly the "blade," [which represents] the power over, the power to dominate,

and destroy and kill. That is a kind of power. But there's also the power of the "chalice," the power to give life, to nurture life. Living a nurturing life has not been considered appropriate for men, so we do have to pay attention at this point still to stereotypes of what's masculine and what's feminine.

Why did dominator cultures start? Is there one thing that can explain it?

Riane: There are many theories. Cross-cultural data, like surveys on where male dominance predominates, found that the more male-dominated cultures were in environments of scarcity. There was more of a tendency to develop the dominator model in areas where the earth was not a good mother, whereas in the more fertile, more life-supporting areas there was more of a tendency towards the partnership model. I think that the domination model really is characterized by scarcity, and it isn't just material scarcity by hoarding by those on top—or the destructiveness of warfare, but also the emotional scarcity of caring.

Why are women controlled because of scarcity?

Riane: To begin with, women are unpaid labor in the dominator model. They are possessions and their children are, as well. I think one of the pieces is trauma. From my work on brain neurochemistry I know traumatized individuals go very much into fight or flight. So institutionalized trauma, from scarcity of safety is one thing for children, it's perpetual, it's the system.

Where do you think the fear of female sexuality comes from?

Riane: I'm not sure that it's a fear. I think it's more a desire to control. Men are not naturally afraid of women, but it's all part of the domination model. And women of course do let out, if I may just say this, a lot of their pent-up frustration in rigidly male-dominated societies on the only male they can, their sons. So it feeds. Women become agents of the system. That's why I always say it's not a question of the women against men or the men against women, it's a question of people doing what they're taught to do. The first president of Kenya insisted that genital mutilation was the most important Kenyan tradition. They've changed now, though.

A lot of the Old Testament is about God being angry that the people—men and women—backslid into Goddess worship, because they thought life was better when they worshipped Her.
Riane: That's right. There was prosperity and peace. The wives baked cakes for the Queen of Heaven and the women were the priestesses, offering the sacred bread, the sacred cake rather than the burnt offering, the sacrifice.

Do you have any thoughts on the suggestion that Jesus and Mary Magdalene were married?
Riane: To me the significant thing isn't whether they were husband and wife, and had children, to me the significant thing is that she really had the powers of a priestess. And that so much of some of the Gnostic belief system reinstated the image of god as mother and the feminine power so that women could baptize in the early Christian communities. And again what it tells me is that we've been robbed of our real history and the history that shows women their power.

As a Holocaust survivor, how did you come to your ideas and how do you define your faith now?
Riane: Having witnessed so much brutality and having learned that almost everybody in my family got wiped out, got murdered, having seen my father pushed down the stairs by the Nazis, and also having seen my mother display what I call spiritual courage, the courage not to kill, to stand up against injustice and risk her life. I really needed to know what is it that makes it possible for people to be so cruel? And does it have to be this way or are there alternatives? I didn't find answers in the conventional studies, about the role of the social system, the partnership and domination models.

My faith right now, I would say, for the last twenty-five years has really been in the life force—in the powers that give life and pleasure and health and joy. And that's in us. There just has to be an energy force that we are blessed to carry and which even has neurochemical rewards of pleasure for when we are caring. I'll tell you the truth. I pray when I'm scared. *[laughter]* I spend a lot of my time being grateful and that's a kind of a constant prayer.

What's your practical advice to women?

Riane: First of all, work on empowering women, because if you work to empower women worldwide, you're empowering yourself. You are creating not only opportunities for others, but for yourself and your daughters, and your sons, because only by empowering women can you really change the domination system that threatens us all today. Make your goal that you're going to become actively involved. Find a way to be economically self-sufficient. There ought to also be reciprocity in every relationship as well as some caring for yourself. Try to really give in to yourself in any way that you can. I wrote in *The Power of Partnership*, the Golden Rule was wonderful: do unto others as you would like them to do unto you. But how about doing unto *you [laughter]* as you would like others to do unto you?

One of the best pieces of advice would be don't take so much advice. *[laughter]* Seek in yourselves, try to figure out what has kept you back and realize your authentic voice and seek advice from it.

That may be one of the great challenges for women, because you're not supposed to want, you're not supposed to desire, you're supposed to be desired. You're not supposed to be goal-oriented, our goal is supposed to be the helpmate. Well, we've been really trained for renunciation. Such a huge part of the joy of being human is to desire, to anticipate, to become engaged rather than disengaged. Dominator propaganda tells you, don't worry, it's okay, all you need to do is just sort of detach yourself and renounce any pleasure, joy.

We have a theory that women are evolving emotionally and spiritually and our challenge is more about creating something for the future as opposed to looking back to the past and finding the golden answer.

Riane: I always make that extremely important point. What has been denied to us in the dominator model is the really active participation in the image of the divine and in the role of priestess, which has very, very ancient roots. It's important that we reclaim those roots because we must reclaim that powerful role, that moral authority. I so want us women to be able to recreate what's ours. Our birthright.

One of our goals is to switch the view of women's history from tragic victims who suffered with dignity, to an acknowledgment and celebration of women who lived pleasure-filled, happy lives.
Riane: It's the human impulse to seek pleasure and avoid pain! *[laughter]* Yet here we have a social system that not only makes it so hard to get it, but that actually makes it sound like suffering is sacred. No. Everyone can learn from suffering, but we don't need to create families, workplaces, nations, and tribes that ensure that we're constantly suffering. It's not necessary.

What gives you the most pleasure?
Riane: Living. My work gives me enormous pleasure. My family gives me a lot of pleasure, my husband. I'm very, very blessed in my second marriage. And my children, my grandchildren. The flowers and walking on the beach. Doing good work that I do, not only the thinking and the writing, but knowing that I am engaged passionately.

CHAPTER 6

Understand Our Long, Illustrious Tradition

Pleasure is ancient

HOW MY PARADIGM CHANGED—MARIA

I could call the change in my thinking an accident, but I don't believe in accidents. A few years ago I was in a strange mood, writing an article, feeling depressed. For some reason I did an Amazon.com search for books on the history of evil. I was wondering, where did the idea of evil start? Who invented it? How universal is it? I'm normally not concerned with evil. I believe in goodness and don't do too many naughty things. But that day it was almost as if I were being guided by an unseen force.

Anyway, up on the screen pops *The Woman with the Alabaster Jar* by Margaret Starbird. Why would a tiny little book that reenvisions the life story of Mary Magdalene be classified under evil? Add to cart. The text presents evidence that Magdalene was a priestess rather than a prostitute as taught by most churches, an equal to Jesus who bore him a daughter after his crucifixion. Starbird frequently references another book, *Holy Blood, Holy Grail*, which also argues that Mary bore Jesus' daughter and that the epic search for the Holy Grail was really an allegory for the search for the descendants of Christ, who were also the descendants of King David. (Is that a good thing? I'm not so sure any-more, having read in 1 Samuel 29 that he killed "his ten thousands.") These books led me to many others that also documented the evidence of ancient female-based religions.

One day, I was talking about these books with my friend Cynthia, terrified that she would think me crazy. Soon after, I got an email from her that read: "You must read *The Da Vinci Code* IMMEDIATELY." A number-one best seller, *The Da Vinci Code* is really a Cliff Notes version of women's religious history.

The primary ritual of the female Goddess religion, which thrived before the growth of the patriarchal religions as we know them, was called the sacred marriage. Both a symbolic and sexual joining of a man and a woman, it represented the universal force of fertility and cre-ation, the merging of both male and female energies in partnership and harmony, and the balance and harmony of male and female principles within each person. The Goddess celebrated pleasure.

Goddess worship also involved a symbolic resurrection. Long be-fore the Gospels recorded that Jesus was crucified, died, and rose again after three days, people had celebrated the dying and rising of the moon every month, noticing that there were three days of dark-ness before the return of the new moon. Every year, in autumn, they observed the death of nature, and, in spring, her rebirth. These cycles of life came to be celebrated as the life and death of the Goddess's male consort.

After steeping myself in the history of Goddess cultures, I started reading the Old Testament which now assumed the form of the story written by an ancient warrior tribe's takeover of other people's land and destruction of their worship of the Goddess—Astarte, The Queen of Heaven—in order to justify their dominance, control, and power over the fertile, sensual, strong, and matrilineal, female power. It amounts to a genocide—and a war on pleasure.

I was a little angry. Suddenly I felt as if the veils of illusion had lifted, as if I had discovered all the untruths I had been living with. For a brief moment in my fortieth year I was able to look at the world and life through a totally clear lens.

Even though some men have tried for ten thousand years to erase and destroy the feminine from our lives, she is still right here with us, like a mother who refuses to abandon her children even though she must suffer abuse and degradation. She is with us at Easter in the Easter egg, the ancient symbol of fertility, as well as in the crucifixion and resurrection of Christ. She is with us at Christmas and Hanukkah (the story of which, by the way, is not written in the Old Testament, or even the Apocrypha), celebrating with stars and candles the return of light represented by the winter solstice. She is the Virgin Mary—"Queen of Heaven." She is the Shinto Ameratsu in Japan. She is Esther and the holiday of Purim. She is with us in the sun, moon, air, soil, and the trees—especially the trees. She is the Black Virgin, who lives in the basement of some Catholic churches, the living embodiment today of the female Goddesses going back to even before Isis.

As I discovered our hidden sacred past, I had the unquenchable urge to reread the romance novels I had devoured as a teenager. *Shanna*, by Kathleen Woodiwiss, was my first and favorite. Oh, it was good. Shanna was a bitch who took six hundred pages to come to her senses and Rouark was the hero to end all heroes. Soon I was reading two or three novels a week and beginning to wonder if there was something wrong with me. Why did I, a smart, educated, intellectual, successful, happily married woman crave these stories? I felt ashamed for reading what many colleagues considered formulaic "drivel." I had been taught that women weren't supposed to enjoy sex, but I was enjoying it and the books are filled with it. It came from hearing from the culture around me that smart, "liberated" women are not supposed to believe in romantic true love (but I did). And finally, the shame came from hearing romances made fun of and ridiculed in the classroom, at work, and in magazines I was reading.

Rather than abandon the pleasure, however, I became more and more convinced that there was a reason I was obsessed with these stories. And once I figured it out, I would be free of it. Eventually, I realized that the romance novel "formula"—the uniting of a man and woman, transformed by love—is a manifestation of the Sacred Marriage in modern times. I find it enormously reassuring that millions of women are secretly (it's still shameful to read romances in public) seeking and worshiping that primal need to love, to heal through love, and to balance the male and female in themselves and their lives.

Dear Reader, you have to understand the extent of this need for love—romance novels are the largest-selling genre of all books in the world. They succeed without critical or intellectual acceptance, without being promoted in mainstream media, without being socially acceptable to read. Women in both red and blue states read them voraciously. We read them because we have an innate desire for love and, deep in our ancient souls, we remember and understand that the transformational power of love is the secret to saving the world. We believe that great sex is important, too.

I wish I could remember the exact moment when I realized the connection between romances and Goddess worship, but it just creeped up on me after the two-hundredth or so romance novel and the twentieth or so book on religious and women's history. Now, this belief is just part of who I am. Now I see myself as part of a long, ancient, and wonderful tradition that has been suppressed, but is like the wild weed that, when cut back, will not die, but rises again and again because its roots are so deep. The plant that grows from this stubborn, tenacious root is pleasure, and the seeds it spreads are the seeds of love.

Religion, like life, is about evolution. It's up to us women to create the new future—a new idea of God—and the only thing worth basing it on is Love.

> *Those men, envious and anxious, not only fired the great*
> *goddess . . . but they also spent thousands of years and billions*
> *of dollars trying to conceal the fact of her existence.*
> —TOM ROBBINS, SKINNY LEGS AND ALL

TAKING OFF THE CORSET—MAYA

At one time, I actually agreed that the absence of women from my history textbook was unremarkable. Now, I don't know which is more appalling—the fact that I thought that, or the fact that no one in my history class had an inkling that there was more to the history of women than prostitution, corsets, and child rearing.

Women's history doesn't lie in the dates of historic events. It lives within the ballrooms of a romance novel, the architecture of a cathedral, the pages of literature, and the swish of crinoline skirts. I've now done my fair share of reading up on women's history that wasn't taught in school. I discovered powerful, determined women who thought, acted, and contributed to our cultural story. But I decided, in the name of research, to try to experience what it was like for the women who had paved the way for us. So, I put on a corset and went to church.

The corset and the Church have long been accused of oppressing women. Yet according to my readings, women were in favor of wearing it, despite (correct) warnings from their (male) doctors about the dangers it posed to their health. In fact, the corset felt kind of good, supportive, giving me phenomenal cleavage. And it kept me from slouching in church, although by lunchtime, I had gotten a little light-headed.

Grace Church, where I went in downtown Manhattan, resembles a small cathedral. Since I seem to be incapable of paying attention during services, I stared at the stained glass windows, the vaulted ceilings, and arches. I was reminded of something I had read in *The Templar Revelation* by Lynn Picknett and Clive Prince: "The great Gothic doorways, through which generations of Christians have passed so innocently, are actually representations of the most intimate parts of the goddess." In other words, those arches with the gigantic rose window at the peak are really supposed to be giant vaginas complete with clitoris. Yes, I was thinking about sex in church, but maybe that's the secret point of the architecture.

The ancient Greek playwright, Euripides, wrote that, "as for the holy rituals performed for the fates and the nameless Goddesses, these are not holy in men's hands; but among women they flourish, every one of them. Thus in holy service woman plays the righteous role." No matter how repressed women were in classical Greek society, religion was their respected domain. I had also read that the gowns and robes that priests wear are like the dresses of the ancient priestesses, adopted as a way to cop some of the priestesses' magical religious powers, since another ancient Greek philosopher wrote "religion only works when in the hands of the females." Alone in my pew, I sat in the light of a stained glass window that depicted not one, but four Marys: the Virgin, the Magdalene, Mary of Bethany, and another Mary I had never heard of. These Marys had had front row seats at the foundation of the Church and were eyewitnesses to the resurrection. They also have their own gospels, which were suppressed but are now being redis-covered.

After church, I went to the Metropolitan Museum of Art, pretending

I had a chaperone, because for most of history a woman of marriageable age would not have been allowed to go on outings alone (although at my age, twenty-two, I'd qualify as an on-the-shelf spinster). There, I took my time in the *Dangerous Liaisons* exhibit: models in eighteenth century period dress, corsets and sparkling jewels, frozen in compromising positions in recreated ballrooms complete with chandeliers. I wandered through the rest of the museum, stopping to admire portraits of wives of great men. In the portrait of Madame and Monsieur Lavoisier painted by the neoclassical painter Jacques-Louis David in 1788, the husband stares adoringly at his wife but she stares out at the viewer. In one tiny room, two paintings seemed to say it all. One, simply titled "An Anonymous Woman," depicted a wife, with every inch but her face and hands covered by corset and fabric. On the opposite wall, a naked woman struck a Vogue-worthy pose as Diana the huntress, bow and arrow in hand.

There are layers of meaning to every painting, every piece of architecture, every ancient story. To gain real understanding, we have to strip away surfaces and most customary views to reveal the truths that lie underneath. And there is nothing as pleasurable as removing a corset and taking a full, unrestrained, deep breath.

Women did indeed do many amazing, heroic things that didn't involve housekeeping. Even if what they did was cook and clean and go to church in a corset, those functions kept the world together, and they were important. Until recently, women's history, both adventurous and domestic, has been invisible. But just because our history isn't told in the history 101 textbooks doesn't mean it doesn't exist.

Discover your history. Billions of women worked hard and took chances and suffered to get where we are today. They would be proud of us. Live the life you want, because you can, and because most of our ancestors couldn't.

DO IT: DELVE INTO OUR COMMON HISTORY

Do your own research. It may seem like hard work, since you have to dig deeper than usual. And don't be surprised if you get angry when you read some of what has been hidden. But sometimes the greatest pleasure comes after you've made the greatest effort.

Much of the evidence for our feminine history has only come to light in the last fifty years as women have become archeologists, scientists, and historians. And some of it continues to be suppressed because of the uninhibited sexual nature of the old goddess culture. A recent *New York Times* article, for example, on sexual behavior research in academia states that, "Decades after the sexual revolution, sex researchers in the United States still operate in a kind of scientific underground, fearing suppression or public censure" from conservative politicians who control government funding, and religious watch groups that actually create lists of academic offenders. Only a few colleges and universities have women's studies programs rather than token courses. Educated women have indeed become dangerous to the male world order, since as we learn, explore, discover, and remember our history and how we got here, it's like waking up from a long, crazy dream and regaining our power.

Here are a few books on women's history that we recommend:

Who Cooked the Last Supper? Rosalind Miles

The Chalice and the Blade and *Sacred Pleasure*, Riane Eisler

Jesus and the Lost Goddess, Timothy Freke and Peter Gandy

When God Was a Woman, Merlin Stone

If you are brave enough to tackle reading the *Old Testament*, buy an ecumenical copy such as the *New Oxford Annotated Bible*. The footnotes and chapter introductions are helpful in seeing the book in its historical context.

LIST: SEEING OUR HOLIDAYS IN A NEW LIGHT*

Most major religious holidays were based on early pagan (pre-Judeo-Christian) holidays that were just too popular to be ignored when the dominant religions took over and established the yearly calendar. *Pagan*, by the way, originally meant "country-dweller" or peasant. So the new authorities kept the dates but changed the stories a little bit, until years later the original cause for celebration was mostly forgotten. Yet it is

* All of this information is from *The Women's Encyclopedia of Myths and Secrets*, by Barbara G. Walker [San Francisco: Harper, 1983].

good to know that certain days and times of year are still kept sacred as the Goddess liked, even if the reason changed. It gives us a sense of connection to our ancestors.

Christmas: Christmas day wasn't designated as Jesus' birthday until three hundred years after his death. If you think the church in Jerusalem might have had some record of his birth to confirm it, think again. That church didn't start celebrating Christmas until the seventh century. And still not every Christian church agrees. The Greek Orthodox church celebrates the birth of Jesus during Twelfth Night, or the Epiphany, which is based on the Alexandrian holiday when the divine Virgin Kore gave birth to the new Aeon (or year). Romans favored December 25, since it was also the birthday of "the unconquered sun," which honored the gods Attis, Dionysus, Osiris, and Baal. Pagans celebrated the birth of a divine child during winter solstice (named Adonis, Tammuz, Joshua, Jehu, among others). The practice of having a decorated tree and gifts, lights, carols, feasts, and processions has pagan origins. Christmas trees evolved from the practice of Roman priests cutting a pine tree from pine groves attached to the temples of the Great Mother the night before a holy day.

When the Puritans came to Massachusetts, they tried to ban Christmas completely, since it was such a pagan holiday. They failed.

Easter: Determined by the lunar calendar (it's the first Sunday after the first full moon after the spring equinox), this sacrificial holiday is for the goddess Eostre (one of the names of the great Goddess, and the northern version of Astarte). The holiday celebrates the seasonal rebirth of nature, plants coming back to life in spring after winter. The rabbit (Easter bunny), older than Christianity, was the moon-hare, sacred to the Goddess. The Easter egg originally symbolized rebirth and was usually colored red, the color of blood. Overall, Easter is a holiday of death and rebirth. The idea of Jesus' death and resurrection is not far off from its origins in myths of Osiris, Dionysus, Demeter, and Persephone.

The Jewish equivalent of Easter is Purim, named after Queen Esther (Esther/Easter!). It is the only Jewish holiday inspired by a woman, and is actually based on a popular pre-Jewish (Goddess) holiday.

As a culture and as individuals, we have *evolved*. We know so much more now about the universe, our own bodies and how they work, about our environment. But we also need to learn and remember the root of our current practices, to awaken our own will to determine our own future. There are lots more ancient stories just waiting for you to seek and find them.

IN HER OWN VOICE: MARY MAGDALENE

"And the companion of the Savior is Mary Magdalene. But Christ loved her more than all the disciples and used to kiss her often on her mouth. The rest of the disciples were offended by it and expressed disapproval. They said unto him, 'Why do you love her more than all of us?' The Savior answered and said to them, 'Why do I not love you like her?' When a blind man and one who sees are both together in darkness, they are no different from one another. When the light comes, then he who sees will see the light, and he who is blind will remain in darkness."

THE GOSPEL OF PHILIP, THE GNOSTIC TEXT—A.D. 350

"Then Peter said to him, 'You have been explaining every topic to us; tell us one other thing. What is the sin of the world?'

The Savior replied, 'There is no such thing as sin; rather you yourselves are what produces sin when you act in accordance with the nature of adultery, which is called "sin." For this reason, the Good came among you, pursuing (the good) which belongs to every nature. It will set it within its root.'

Then he continued. He said, 'This is why you get sick and die: because [you love] what deceives you. [Anyone who] thinks should consider (these matters)!

"That is why I told you, 'Become content at heart, while also remaining discontent and disobedient; indeed become contented and agreeable (only) in the presence of that other Image of nature."

"Aquire my peace within yourselves! Be on your guard so that no one deceives you by saying, 'Look over here!' or 'Look over there!' For the child of true Humanity exists within you. Follow it! Those who search for it will find it."

THE GOSPEL OF MARY MAGDALENE—A.D. 150

PLEASURE REVOLUTIONARY: MARY MAGDALENE

In the late sixth century Pope Gregory "the Great" (that bastard!) declared Mary Magdalene a whore. His declaration had nothing to do with the account that Jesus kissed her on the mouth, since the *Gospel of Thomas* was hidden in a jar in a cave and wouldn't be found until 1945. But it had everything to do with the misogyny of the Church. Mary was clearly a powerful woman in the Bible—if you read it yourself you can see that—but reading the Bible yourself was punishable by death until after the Protestant Reformation in the 1500s. What could the Church authorities have been trying to hide? Mary is mentioned in the gospels of Matthew, Luke, Mark, and John as being the first to see the risen Christ. And even St. Augustine, renowned misogynist, called her "the apostle to the apostles."

The Bible does not record that Mary was a prostitute. It does say Jesus cast out seven demons from her. Healing practices at the time also considered that a sick person was "possessed" and had to be exorcised to be healed. The seven demons are often interpreted to be the "seven sins," although there is no evidence to support that. She might just have been depressed. It may be a coincidence that, "The cult of Ishtar or Astarte—the mother goddess and 'Queen of Heaven'—involved, for example, a seven-stage initiation," according to the authors of *Holy Blood, Holy Grail.*

Some historians and theologians believe that Mary was the wife of Jesus, or a priestess. In *The New Testament*, a number of Marys act in wifely or priestess-like ways, but none can be proven to be the same Mary as the Madgalene. But, in those times, it was rare for any man to have so many women publicly associate with him. A footnote in the *New Oxford Annotated Bible* states that, "Given ancient Palestinian attitudes toward women, this association of the Galilean women with Jesus' ministry is remarkable, as is the mixture of the sexes among the followers."

In the early 1900s, the Gnostic Gospels were discovered in Nag Hammadi, and *The Gospel of Mary* was found by an antique dealer in Germany. Both were published in translation in the mid 1900s, and are considered by a majority of historians to be authentic and significant for their additional and sometimes alternative views of Biblical events.

The Gospel of Mary is only a few pages long (many pages are missing), but offers insight into Mary and the early apostles. Karen King, a professor at Harvard Divinity School, writes in her introduction to *The Gospel of Mary of Magdala*, "This astonishingly brief narrative presents a radical interpretation of Jesus' teachings as a path to inner spiritual knowledge; it rejects his suffering and death as the path to eternal life; it exposes the erroneous view that Mary of Magdala was a prostitute for what it is—a piece of theological fiction; it presents the most straight-forward and convincing argument in any early Christian writing for the legitimacy of women's leadership; it offers a sharp critique of illegiti-mate power and a utopian vision of spiritual perfection; it challenges our rather romantic views about the harmony and unanimity of the first Christians; and it asks us to rethink the basis for church authority. All written in the name of a woman."

One consistent theme in *The Gospel of Mary*, *The Gospel of Philip*, and *The Gospel of Thomas* is the animosity that Peter, considered the founder of the Christian church, has for Mary. Levi, a follower of Jesus, calls him a "hot-head" because Peter doesn't believe that Jesus would have chosen her to speak with about anything privately or, as the Greek version reads: "Surely he [Jesus] didn't want to show that she is more worthy than *we* are?" Levi replies: "Assuredly the Savior's knowl-edge of her is completely reliable. That is why he loved her more than us." In the end, Peter's faction won out and Gospels that were contrary to his misogynistic view were edited out. Fortunately, a few copies were hidden—to be found 1,500 years later.

Holy Blood, Holy Grail, made famous by *The Da Vinci Code*, makes the case that Mary escaped to France after the crucifixion and bore Jesus a daughter, literally embodying the "Holy Grail" or *sang real* (literal translation: holy blood) that has obsessed people for millennia. The purpose of maintaining the lineage of Mary and Jesus seems to be more about protecting the royal line of King David than it is to con-tinue the teachings that are more self-directed and inner-directed than the institutional church feels comfortable with. The authors build a strong case that she is the mother of the Merovingian dynasty, which ruled France in the Middle Ages. They also make the case that Mary Magdalene is the "our lady" behind all the French Notre Dames—not the Blessed Virgin Mary.

The Magdalene is often symbolized by the Black Virgin or Madonna, which also represents the long lineage of female deities before her—from the Egyptian Isis to the Hindu Kali, to Astarte and all the other Queens of Heaven before her. What we find especially wonderful about the Black Virgin is that DNA analysis has shown that we actually have all descended from one black woman in Africa.

Ultimately, it doesn't matter if Mary had sex with Jesus, if she was married to him or not, or even if she bore any of his children. What matters is that all the evidence shows that she was loved and respected by Jesus. And he would probably be justifiably angry to know that representatives of a church founded on his name were calling her a whore.

CHAPTER 7

Enjoy Your Body

Pleasure starts inside of you

FROM SHAME AND GUILT TO ACCEPTANCE—MARIA

I still remember the joy of going shirtless as a child. In the hot summer, I exposed my bare skin to fresh air. No shame. No self-consciousness. Then the shame about my female body started. Perhaps initiated by a few scolds that adults thought appropriate, and probably a few teases from siblings or neighbors. But it also came from reading body language and signals around me: the pinched, disapproving look on people's faces when I asked certain questions about sex or said certain things about my body, the lack of discussion of the changes going on in my and my sister's bodies.

Around the time when my sexuality started to bubble and froth, I noticed that it was considered secret, dark, shameful, even sinful. We in our family didn't talk about it. But, being curious, I explored, experimented, and tried to understand my body. I started to feel guilt when it seemed that no one else had these feelings, these problems. The main message I got from the people around me, and the culture, was that it was wrong to have them.

When I finally blossomed into a lovely young woman, I was totally unprepared to deal with the swarm of taunting, flirting, tempting men who swarmed me like flies. I actually thought that they liked me for my sparkling personality and sharp mind instead of my budding breasts. My self-esteem was inappropriately bolstered by their attentions. It took me years of mistakes to finally realize that my body is my own. I am responsible for it. And there is nothing shameful or guilty about loving it.

It's ironic to me that when I had the beauty of youth, I didn't get much pleasure from my body. But now that I'm in my forties, I know what I like and what I don't like and I don't feel shame or guilt about either my body or my desires. I've got my maternal grandmother's double chin, and both grandmothers' beefy Eastern European upper arms. I have my Mother's belly, both parents' frizzy hair, and my boobs are dropping fast. My body is not pleasing by contemporary fashion terms. I'm curvy, short, and plump—more like an old fashioned painting. So it's often hard for me to find clothes that fit, or feel good about myself in them, especially when I'm on TV next to dyed and dolled-up pencil-thin celebrities.

But I love my body. I've learned to love it. I've studied it like a difficult work of literature that needs time and seasoning to be truly understood. Plus, I'm kind of proud of it. Even after giving birth to two children and miscarrying three I can stand on my head, do a cartwheel, jump on the giant trampoline, and find lots and lots of physical pleasure—without shame or guilt (or I wouldn't be telling you about it!).

I've been able to do this because I've really examined shame and guilt and where it comes from. In a way, that's what this book is truly about. Cultures that are largely controlled by men try to stifle and control female sexuality as much as possible, knowing they need to implant their seed in us in order to have heirs. Sexuality is such a primal survival and evolutionary force that it cannot be stopped (without stopping the world). So male authorities created the virgin/whore dichotomy: virgins are for wives, whores are for pleasure. Virgins go to heaven, whores go to hell, and the men don't worry because God is on their side. When cultures and men try to suppress sexuality, it comes out in all sorts of ugly ways—priests abusing children, men raping women, women abusing their own bodies. Even today in many cultures, women are conditioned to believe that if they really, truly enjoy sex then they are sluts.

Reading romances helped me come to terms with my sexuality and my own pleasure. Many romances are filled with hot sex. Even our agent admitted after we made her read a romance novel that it was hotter than most erotica she has read. Millions of women in jeans and sweatshirts on their weekly food-shopping trip are adding some real spice to their carts—and their lives. Don't tell Walmart.

We all want sex. Even if we say we don't, we do. But we want sex with pleasure. We don't want to be forced or used. We don't want to be taken without being given back to. We want our partner to consider our pleasure—physical, emotional, and spiritual. We want the sex to be almost sacred, like it used to be before they tried to confuse us. And sometimes we do want it hot and thrilling. Why should I—or you—feel guilty or ashamed about that?

BODILY FICTIONS—MAYA

I once took a class called "Bodily Fictions," which was about how the media messes up women's expectations of what our bodies should look like. To promote class discussion, the teacher showed us fashion advertisements. While everyone in the class—about twenty girls and one gay guy—bitched about the symbolism, repression, and unrealistic expectations, I just wanted to know where I could get that bathing suit, because I never really had body image problems.

Sure, there are things I don't like—for example, all the scars from every mosquito bite that I couldn't resist scratching. And my legs are kind of bowed. I get pimples. But for the most part, my body is quite all right. It's mine and it works and that's more important to me than anything else.

"Bodily Fictions" made me so irritated and angry that I had to drop it. I wanted an educational experience, not a therapy group. I believe enjoyment of your body is up to you—feeling bad about yourself because of an airbrushed model isn't anyone else's fault but your own. But I've been exposed to certain attitudes and images that contributed to my confidence.

When I was about eight years old, my mom took me to see a foreign movie called *Like Water for Chocolate*, about food and sex and love. There were a lot of naked people in it. I was mildly scandalized. In fact, it kind of freaked me out, but I bragged to my friends how liberal my mom was. I saw the movie again when I was seventeen and it wasn't as naked as I thought. But when I was in the dark movie theatre seeing a naked man for the first time, and a naked girl with this man for the first time, and a naked woman riding a horse through the Mexican desert, I was a little uncomfortable, but my mom acted like it was all OK. She didn't shield my eyes, or demand we leave, or say that nudity was wrong, sinful, or shameful. To her credit, the movie wasn't rated, but it was that sort of nonchalance that said to me that naked bodies and using them as an expression of love was cool.

When I was nineteen, I spent the summer in Paris and took a class on French art in the eighteenth and nineteenth centuries, which seemed more like a class in "Portraits of Naked Women." Every afternoon, in a dark classroom, we would look at slides of naked women in various poses, most often bathing. Slide after slide of naked women bathing, or brushing their hair, or lounging around flashed up on the screen. They all blended together until Manet's *Olympia* popped up. It is a portrait of a prostitute, posing as a prostitute, naked, with one little hand covering up the area between her legs. In the background is a dark woman bringing in a bouquet of flowers, presumably from a suitor. A black cat on the bed arches its back, tail erect. When first exhibited in the Parisian Salon, the painting caused a huge scandal, perhaps because Manet ignored the tradition that female nudity was only acceptable if she was posing as a goddess, or perhaps because most of the men viewing the painting with their wives had tasted the talents of the subject. Perhaps it is because of The Look on Olympia's face as she gazed out at the viewer, one that seemed to say, "I am naked and I am not ashamed."

We visited Olympia in the Musée D'Orsay. Seeing it at a time when I was getting naked with boys for the first time was a blessing. I had also seen the magazine photo spreads and advertisements that seemed to induce self-loathing and eating disorders in many girls, but those weren't hanging in museums, being talked about hundreds of years later. I made my choice. Being naked and not having issues with my body was just more fun.

The real test of comfort was posing for a full-length nude portrait for my boyfriend, who is a painter. He needed a model and I volunteered. I had my reservations, but I was drawn to the idea of a lasting image of my beautiful body. The difficult part was not having him stare at me for hours on end—in fact, I enjoyed that aspect—but standing still on a chair for an extended amount of time. I thought of the look on Olympia's face, and hoped that the same confidence came through in my posture and expression. Every twenty minutes we would take a break, and drink some absinthe and talk. I imagined this is what life was like for the artists in Paris at the turn of the twentieth century. It felt like we were actively participating in a long and glorious tradition.

It's not the advertising guys, or the models, or movies, or paintings that make you feel bad about your naked self. They shouldn't make you feel good about it either. Seeing positive portrayals of women and their bodies is very important, it has helped me, but only so much. At some point, it's just up to you to say, "This is me. I like me. My body does amazing things for me." It's up to you to be like Olympia, to stare out and say, "I am naked, and I like it. Got a problem with it?"

DO IT: SLEEP NAKED

Surprisingly, according to all the research we've read, only a minority of men and women sleep naked. This surprises us, since sleeping naked on good sheets is one of our greatest pleasures.

Sleeping naked means that there is nothing between you and the sheets to attempt to choke, squeeze, or chafe you while you fall blissfully into slumber. Sleeping naked means that you and your body are alone together for the whole night, reveling in freedom and unfettered rest.

Sleeping naked is not about sex, really, or looking sexy. Sleeping naked is about being you and you alone. Maybe it's a bit about going back to the womb, before onesies and diapers, and shame and tags that scratch, back to when you were surrounded by the warmth and loving embrace of a mysterious mother you had yet to meet, but knew in your soul.

SHEET TIPS FOR SLEEPING NAKED

Satin is slippery, but nice. Flannel is warm and soft when it's new, but as it gets washed it gets nubby and rough. Cheap sheets can give you brush burns. The higher the thread count, the softer and more delightful the sheets will feel. Cotton Jersey sheets are very soft and smooth.

Organic cotton helps you sleep with a clean conscience. Layer lots of pads—feather, sheepskin, or cotton—between your mattress and your sheets for cloud-like slumber.

LIST: BIZARRE BODY CUSTOMS FROM AROUND THE WORLD

Foot binding: China—Brace yourself, ladies. Imagine breaking your little three-year-old daughter's toes, folding them under, and wrapping them up forever. Then when she's a bit older, perhaps six, break her arch. Foot binding was done to keep girls from going anywhere. She could not have been married without having totally nonfunctioning "lily feet." The practice is believed to have started because of some prince's foot fetish in the tenth century B.C., yet it wasn't outlawed until 1911 . . . almost three thousand years later.

Neck elongation: Burma—A long graceful neck is beautiful, so an even longer neck must be ideal, right? Tradition says that it was begun to protect the women's necks from tiger attacks. But it is also said that if a woman is caught "straying" the husband has the right to remove the necklaces. Unfortunately, her neck is no longer able to hold her head up and folds over, leading to asphyxiation.

Clitoridectomies: Africa and some Middle Eastern countries— Sometimes removal of the clitoris is done to infants, but mostly it's done to young girls between the ages of four and eight (before they are old enough to understand and rebel). Thank goodness, girls and their mothers are starting to resist. And while it's tempting to blame one of the misogynistic religions, the practice actually predates them. Generally, in a clitoridectomy, the girl is held down by the women she has known and loved. With no anesthesia, her clitoris is removed using a shard of glass, a tin lid, or a rusty old knife. Sometimes her whole labia are removed, too, and her vagina sewn up leaving a teeny hole barely big enough to let out urine and menstrual blood. The practice makes the vagina nice and tight for their husbands, and ensures the woman feels no pleasure from sex. In fact, for her wedding night her vagina is often torn open and sewn back up again the next day. The women be-lieve that a clitoridectomy is essential to their health. Some even believe that a clitoris is dangerous and if it accidentally touches a man's penis or a baby's head during childbirth it will kill the man or baby. It's a savage custom, but every day six thousand little girls have it done to them. More than 140 million women are walking around (painfully) today who have had this done to them.

America had its own phase of clitoridectomies. In the early 1800s women's organs were seen as the origins of most behavioral problems in women, and anesthesia made it safe to remove them. More than 150,000 women had their ovaries removed to make them more orderly and "cleanly." According to Gail Collins in *America's Women:* "Physicians did not believe that even very young girls minded being deprived of their clitoris or ovaries. 'We must not impute to a woman feelings in regard to the loss of her organs which are derived from what we as men would think of a similar operation on a man. A woman does not feel she is unsexed, and she is not unsexed,' Dr. Cushing counseled his fellow physicians." Even twenty years ago, women were told to get unnecessary hysterectomies after having their last child, because physicians were taught that the uterus was for growing babies or growing cancer.

Veiling of women: Middle East/Islamic countries—In some countries the veil is called the burqa and in others the chador. Used as a status symbol among upper classes, the veil predates Islam, and is less about God and modesty than it is about fashion. The use of the veil protects a woman's mystery and represents the belief that men can't be trusted to control themselves around any part of a woman's body—even an exposed wrist. It wasn't until two hundred years after Mohammed that the veil became commonplace, but many Middle Eastern women choose to see it as part of their ancient culture, which, as an old saying goes, believes that "a woman belongs in the house—or in a grave." It is also seen as a political statement in support of the conservative practice of Islam. In the most conservative Islamic countries, women don't have a choice about veiling themselves, and face brutal treatment if they dare show their face in public.

Breast implants: America—Yes, we use anesthesia and surgically sterile instruments, but the primal urge is to enhance our attractiveness to the opposite sex, whether or not it gives us any more pleasure, whether or not it makes us sick, whether or not it actually makes us look any better.

Remember ladies, the majority of these practices are performed and perpetuated by women, mother to daughter, grandmother to granddaughter. You can choose to end the cycle of suffering.

IN HER OWN VOICE: EVE ENSLER

"I was drawn to vaginas because of my own personal history, because of sexuality, because women's empowerment is deeply connected to their sexuality."

"I've been an activist my whole life, and I was active for a lot of different issues. But four years ago, I made a commitment to devote the rest of my life to ending violence towards women. And that has shifted everything. Now everything's lined up. There's a right order, right relationship. There's clarity."

"I feel . . . that I'm inside my vagina for the first time in my life . . . I'm in my life. I'm in my seat. I'm in my core. I'm in my power. I don't feel apologetic about anything anymore. I feel a determination I've never felt before in my life. And the possibility of really, really impacting and changing things—that, in fact, we could create a world where women could live safely and freely without being abused or raped. Talking about vaginas all the time has given me that confidence and strength."

PLEASURE REVOLUTIONARY: EVE ENSLER—
THE VAGINA LADY

Thanks to Eve Ensler, vagina is no longer a dirty word. In fact, thanks to Eve Ensler, you can actually say the word vagina out loud. An interest in women's empowerment and sexuality, as well as rape, violence, and incest led Eve to that certain part of female anatomy. She started talking to friends about the vagina in general, their perceptions of it, and attitudes toward it. Eventually, she interviewed two hundred women, just talking about their vaginas. And those conversations gave birth to the play *The Vagina Monologues*, for which the phrase enormous success might be an understatement. It won an Obie Award, has been translated into more than thirty-five languages, and is running

hemselves. In her own life she has transcended
g her hurt into a positive force, and even work-
tionship with her mother. She is an inspiration
orks relentlessly to make sure no other women
rating women and their bodies, and in her work
iolence against women, Eve makes the world safer,
more accessible for women and their vaginas.

in theaters all over th
day, celebrated or
purpose is cle

Her 1-
the boo,
in women
bodies in or
finally on goo
no longer flat. An
ach and body turne
diverse women, quest.
the self-loathing that oi
her body, she says, "I thin
we've been taught and traine
and mutilating ourselves. That
have power in the world. It's this h
path. The only way you can undo it
the obsession of it."

Her work to change the violent circu.
may be due to her own childhood experience.
physical abuse by her father. The sexual abuse e
years old and went undetected by her mother, bt
continued. As a high school student, she was "self-mt
cohol. She attended college at Middlebury College ii.
was accepted to Yale Drama School, but couldn't afford
she was twenty-four, she stopped drinking and started writ.
theater.

The recipient of a Guggenheim Fellowship Award for playwi.
as well as numerous others, Eve is first a playwright, but her work n
involves a lot more activism in bringing attention to her V-Day cause.
Whether V is for Vagina or Vote, Eve's work brings women and their
bodies positive attention and respect. For the future she says, "I hope
the next stage of V-Day is that women choose to be great instead of
good. That would mean living with ambiguity, living with not being
approved of, living with your voice, living with your originality, living
with the mess and living with your power."

Eve Ensler is a pleasure revolutionary for making it OK to talk
about vaginas, taking away any shame, mystery, and locked-up feelings

84

WHAT'S YOUR P
women have had toward t
the cycle of abuse, turnii
ing on healing her rela
for victims, and also
should suffer. In cele
with V-Day to end
and makes pleasur

CHAPTER 8

Find Your Voice

Pleasure knows that good girls speak up

THE VOICE OF SOBRIETY—MARIA

My siblings and I grew up with one main message: "Be nice." But, as in all families and cultures, there were unspoken rules, which I learned by watching. One was, "when you drink, you can do or say anything you want." During the day we were proper, silent, suffering, and polite. But once cocktail hour hit—all bets were off. Sometimes the drinking would lead to rip-roaring good times. Sometimes it would lead to long, rambling speeches. Sometimes, it would lead to pity parties. As an alcohol interventionist I have met described it, "poor me, poor me, pour me another drink."

Then we kids, too, learned to drink. Drinking became our new common bond with my parents. As early as age fourteen, I was allowed with my older brother to sit with my mother after dinner and pound back crème de menthes or Cointreaus. Her verbal justification was "Well, they let the kids drink early in Europe," but we knew she was happy that we were now on her side. When we were drunk we could be as mean as we wanted and we all found it hysterically funny. And the sugary taste was easy to swallow— especially as we usually skipped dessert, because *that* wasn't healthy..

I continued to drink. I drank through high school. Through college, when I drank a lot at home because it was better than getting a babysitter for Maya. I drank my way up the ladder at work—keeping pace with the Guys and the Girl Guys. There, the rules were the same as at home. Keep your mouth shut and be stoic during the day, but once the weaklings leave the bar you can rant and rage and say anything you want. And the best part of it is you hardly remember it in the morning. In later years, I drank a lot with my father—appreciating the unique vein-tingling power of a good red wine. He collected wine and had a wine cellar, filled with the good stuff. I remember how strongly feminist I felt when I learned how to open Champagne bottles myself, which felt like I was proving to him I really was capable.

My father's and brother's deaths worsened my drinking—even though they had been my best drinking buddies. My mother called their funerals "celebrations of life" and wanted a positive face kept on the whole thing. But I did not really feel like celebrating. Our grief was jammed deep down into our private lives, not shared.

On and off throughout the years I had given up drinking for a year, just to prove I could. I kept thinking that when I started up again I'd finally be able to control myself—to stop properly after the second glass of wine or vodka. It never happened.

It wasn't until Maya turned fourteen that I started to realize the horror of it all. I couldn't believe that my mother had let me drink with her at that young age. My precious Maya wasn't an innocent, but I certainly wouldn't let her drink. I started to be really angry about that part of my childhood and grieve for my own lost innocence. If I hadn't had been drinking so much, maybe I wouldn't have ended up in so many unwanted back seats and basements doing stuff that no amount of drinking could ever erase.

My final night of drinking was at Maya's school fundraising auction—a black tie dinner. For some reason, I just wanted to submerge myself in alcohol. I kept returning to the bar to refill my vodka tonic. I had seven of them. They were going down like sweet fire, seeping into my veins like morphine. From all accounts, I held it together pretty well—even as I spoke with members of the school administration and Maya's friends, who were volunteering that night. But in the car going home I started passing out (thank God, Lou was driving). And the next morning I vomited and vomited. I vowed I would never, ever, drink again. If I couldn't control myself at my own daughter's school, I didn't deserve to drink. My husband wasn't convinced I "never needed to drink again," but I was firm in my resolve.

It's been about six years and a funny thing happened after I stopped drinking. I found my voice.

At first it started coming out kind of like a froggy burp. I'd say things that weren't nice, but were true for me. I couldn't hold back. My family didn't know what to do with me. Then I started a projectile vomiting of rage and defensiveness. I thought that everyone really wanted to hear the truth from me in all its bloody gore. They didn't. Drinking hadn't erased my pain, it had just delayed it. Now I was really feeling it. And I couldn't help but let it out.

Gradually, through lots of coaching and family therapy, I learned how to say what I needed to say without it sounding like a vicious attack. I also learned that all the words in the world won't change other people. What really mattered was my own behavior. But that won't change other people, either.

I finally have been able to create a world around me where I speak the truth as I know it as gently and lovingly as I can, when it truly matters. But I have also learned to speak to stand up for myself and protect myself— whether it's from a teasing comment or a subtle put-down. I've also learned when to walk away.

A lot of people associate pleasure with drinking. But drinking, like sex or food is not inherently evil. It's what people do with it. Some people can handle it. Others can't. It stops being about pleasure when it causes so much pain.

My husband stopped drinking, too. Not because he had the same problems I did with it, but because his religious experience led him to the conclusion that alcohol is a source of suffering in the world. (I had to learn the hard way.) We don't have alcohol in our house. When it came time to hire a new head of our company, I was pleasantly surprised that the two leading candidates didn't drink, either.

Now, whether it's at home or at work, I have a support system around me. We had our fun, but more than ever, we know the complex misery that goes with it. Now, I have a different kind of fun—and in fact I have even more of it. It's good to be sober. It's good to be alive. It's good to wake up each morning clearheaded and guilt free. It's good to have a voice that is now clear and strong. It's especially good to have created a family of my own where we are all free to use our true voices—where no one has to be told to be nice and the sound of laughter rings much more often than the dirge of tears.

SAY WHAT YOU MEAN/MEAN WHAT YOU SAY—MAYA

*Y*our voice is what you say and how you say it. Do you sing it, scream it, whisper it, whine it, write it, ramble on and on about it? And what are you saying, anyway? Most of us just wander around and open our mouths and words fly out. But how we say what we mean—our voice—often reveals much more than the words themselves. Even though eyes are said to be the window to our soul—whoever said that just wanted women to shut up—voices reveal so much more.

I never really noticed all the subtleties a voice could convey until I got a job answering phones as a reservationist for two really popular New York City restaurants. After two years of spending twenty hours a week listening to people ask for the same thing (an eight o'clock reservation), I started listening to *how* they asked, and, in turn, how I responded. Answering phones gets really boring, so I started to make a sort of study to make it bearable.

"Please" goes a long way. "Gimme" does not; neither does calling me "sweetheart," or demanding, "it's going to be at. . . ." Technically, we were obligated to be as accommodating as possible, but one of my co-workers admitted that if she didn't like a person's phone manner then she wouldn't give him a reservation even if it were available. How you say something matters. Exceptions can be made for those who are polite and engaging. Mean, bossy, condescending, irrationally demanding people go hungry, which probably makes them even crankier, but that's a story for another day.

Since I was paid to do things a certain way, I often couldn't really say what I wanted to, so to compensate, I created several tones of voice to express what I could not say in words. By then I had carefully constructed replies down to the intonation of each syllable: "I'm sorry we are fully booked, however . . ." When I had to give a reservation to someone even though I didn't think they deserved it because they were mean (and people can be very mean over the telephone), I used my "seething politeness" voice. I said the right words in a very, very calm manner, laced with venom, that dared them to contradict me—the kind of voice that says, "With one click of a button, I can make this reservation disappear. You wouldn't want me to do that, would you? I thought so." When a person called for the address, I responded in my "listen-carefully-because-I-am-only-going-to-say-this-once" voice. Moms and teachers use this a lot.

That job was more taxing than it may seem. Constantly suppressing what I wanted to say and how I wanted to say it, combined with college writing classes all designed to help me "find my voice" confused and exhausted me. I often bored my friends with work stories about horrible customers, adding in the smart-ass replies I wished I could have said. But this job helped me become aware of when I'm faking my voice, which sometimes it is necessary to do. I learned that a little politeness and understanding goes a long way. I know that customers who threatened and called me names made my heart beat faster with fear, and the next caller may have gotten less than they deserved because of that. I know that my voice affects others, and I want it to affect them in a positive way. Whenever possible, I resort to my old writing mantra: say what you mean and mean what you say. What I mean by that is be honest and be true in the words you use, the feeling behind them, and the way you express them. Sometimes, I was actually sorry that we were fully booked for reservations.

DO IT: CATCH YOURSELF SUBMERGING YOUR VOICE AND THEN SAY IT

It takes time to recognize when you are suppressing your opinion or feelings. The first sign that you are submerging your voice is that you want to tell someone else about it. You have an encounter with someone that you feel you handled politely or respectfully, but then you can't wait to call someone and tell them what you *really* thought and what you *really* wanted to say. Another sign is that you have a bad feeling in your stomach from the encounter. You feel slightly violated, hurt, and confused. You can't sleep because of the conversations you are having in your head. If any of that happens, you know what you have to do.

If you have a drinking problem, there are lots of resources to help.

Call Alcoholics Anonymous. Don't believe for a minute that you are fooling your family and friends. Denial and blaming others are hallmarks of a person with alcohol problems. And you don't need to be a morning drinker to need help.

If someone you love has a problem, read *Love First*, by Jeff Jay and Debra Jay, which explains the intervention process. But know that unless the person is truly ready to make a change, your success may only be temporary. If you grew up with alcoholic parents, read *Adult Children of Alcoholics*, a classic, by Janet Geringer Woititz, Ed.D. It's eye-opening, and will encourage you to stop the cycle that creates a family filled with pain.

LIST: HOW TO EXPRESS YOURSELF SO YOU'LL BE HEARD

Whether you are very angry with someone, or hurt, or in the middle of a horrible conflict—or if you just want to define your boundaries, here are some hard-learned tips on how to express yourself effectively.

Say it (whatever *it* is) in person. For the lord's sake don't write an email or say it over the phone (unless you have absolutely no other choice). When you are face to face with someone, you can see the effect that what you are saying is having on them, and determine if you did it right or not. The other person can see your body language as well.

Use "I" language. Don't say "You never do the dishes and that makes me mad." Say "I really wish that you would do the dishes because I get angry that I have to do them." Saying "you" and accusing people of things immediately puts them on the defensive and they stop listening and caring.

Say it in private. Please, please, please don't say anything hurtful or critical to someone in front of others. We see people all the time scolding, teasing, and insulting one another and it hurts to watch. The humiliation and mortification people feel from being scolded or criticized in public takes years and years to forgive. It never helps your own cause.

Lose the insults. I know one well-meaning parent who screws up his message all the time. He says things like, "I keep telling my son he should go to college . . . *the stupid idiot!*" or, "He's a smart kid, he just doesn't act like it . . . *the knucklehead!*" What do you think the poor kid hears? Never, ever call anyone: stupid, idiot, jerk, or dumb. Those kinds of insults fly back and hit *you* in the eye.

Write the letter, but don't ever send it. It sure feels good to write down your feelings in an uncensored way, doesn't it? Now put it away in a special secret drawer and thank heaven you didn't send it.

Say it with love. This is really hard. Especially if you are really mad. But if you can do this, you can do almost anything.

Sometimes the best response is no response. Some people love to blame, accuse, project anger, and generally try to make your life miserable. Do not, under any circumstances take on their problems and feel guilty for them. Many times their anger is caused by issues, such as substance abuse or trauma, that are out of your control. Giving them attention for their tantrums and outbursts only encourages them to do it even more. In dog training, child rearing, and life, rewarding the good behavior and ignoring the bad behavior is the most effective way to change behavior.

IN HER OWN VOICE: LADY MURASAKI

". . . His Majesty must have had a deep bond with her in past lives as well, for she gave him a wonderfully handsome son. He had the child brought in straightaway, for he was desperate to see him, and he was astonished by his beauty. His elder son, born to his Consort the daughter of the Minister of the right, enjoyed powerful backing and was feted by all as the undoubted future Heir Apparent, but he could not rival his brother in looks, and His Majesty, who still accorded him all due respect, there lavished his private affection on the new arrival."

"He laughed. 'I have been rude and unfair to your romances, haven't I. They have set down and preserved happenings from the age of the gods to our own. *The Chronicles of Japan* and the rest are a mere fragment of the whole truth. It is your romances that fill in the details."

"Murasaki too had become addicted to romances."

TALE OF GENJI, 1972 TRANSLATION

PLEASURE REVOLUTIONARY: LADY MURASAKI—
THE FIRST NOVELIST

The first novelist has one of the most enduring voices in literature, yet we don't even know her real name, although the book is attributed to Shikibu Murasaki. Shikibu is the name of the office her father and elder brother held. Murasaki (which means purple) is a nickname that refers to the main female character in her novel, *The Tale of Genji*. A thousand pages long and written a thousand years ago, it's widely considered to be the first novel ever written. Even after all this time and all the translations, her voice still carries through fresh, female, and formidable.

Murasaki lived about A.D. 973–1020. She was one of those girls who crashed her brother's lessons and was far more intelligent than he. Her father, wishing she had been born a boy so her intelligence wouldn't go to waste, let her have lessons with her brother. After her father was widowed he sent her to the palace of Kyoto to serve as companion to the empress. There she wrote *Genji*. As she finished each chapter, it was passed around the palace and everyone awaited each successive chapter with great anticipation.

During this time, Chinese was the official written language of the Japanese bureaucracy. Women were forbidden to learn it, effectively keeping them out of business and diplomacy. Written Japanese was still being developed—largely by the women who used it for the expression of thoughts and emotions in poems, letters, diaries, and novels, rather than, say, tax laws. Women's writing, and the novel *Genji*, established Japanese literature. As a writer, Murasaki used the language she was permitted to—phonetic Japanese—and molded it, until she had developed a beautiful writing style that conveyed characters who lived long ago, but seem like people we know.

The Tale of Genji is her masterpiece. The novel follows Genji, a court title, not the actual name of the hero (we never know his real name), throughout his life. He is born to an emperor and his beloved intimate, grows up, has dozens of love affairs, breaks hearts, has his heart broken, travels around Japan, meets people and says good-bye. *Genji* depicts the ins and outs of the highly structured Japanese court life, in which nobility and their courtiers spoke and wrote to each other in poetry as a form of competitive creativity. Hundreds of poems appear within the novel.

Murasaki's diary reveals that she had an eye for fashion, and devotes paragraph after paragraph to what people wore and who showed a "want of taste." She had a daughter, but not much is known about her day-to-day life except through her observations, her voice, and her ability to convey sometimes wistful and sometimes cheeky emotions.

In the introduction to the most recent translation, Royall Tyler writes, "Its most celebrated characters live more vividly in the imagination than anyone known from historical documents, and their lives—their sufferings, their disappointments, their failings, and their grace—have remained a major legacy to the centuries that have passed since they were first conceived. Although invented, they are also immortal. Even Genji's Rukujo estate, lovingly reconstructed in drawings and models, is by far the most widely known example of the domestic architecture of its time. That it never existed makes no difference at all."

We can't help but think how much more we would know about life, history, love, and humanity if more women had disobeyed their cultural rules and written down their stories and observations. It would have been better yet if there had been no rules prohibiting women from learning, reading, and writing in the first place. Thankfully, women like Lady Murasaki didn't hold back. She expressed herself. And a millennium later, her voice comes through loud and clear.

CHAPTER 9

Make a List of All the Things You Ever Wanted to Do

Pleasure will take you to unexpected places

STOP WISHING AND START DOING. WHAT DID YOU WANT TO BE WHEN YOU GREW UP?—MARIA

Perhaps being a single parent at the age of twenty made me shunt aside my childhood dreams and focus on how to make a good living. It's not as though I didn't have choices, or even that I regret the choices I made. It was a matter of prioritization. My first job out of college was working for a progressive public relations firm in Washington, D.C. Little Maya and I moved to a one-bedroom apartment downtown and for the first time tasted independence. The independence part was great. The part I didn't like was the negativity. We were anti-nuclear, anti-apartheid, anti-contra, anti–right wing, and definitely anti-Reagan. I asked myself, where can I go to work for a company that is *for* something? At the time, my father was begging me to return to the family business, Maya was ready to enter kindergarten, and I either had to move to a safer neighborhood or do something else for a career. So I went home and got swept up in the family business.

Just before I quit the thankless creative director job, I attended the fateful management retreat where I wrote my own obituary. Given all the deaths of loved ones I had recently experienced, and my own burnt-out, exhausted, and depressed state of being, it didn't seem like such a far-fetched exercise. I wrote something like: "She tried hard to please everyone, but no one was ever quite satisfied—especially herself. She left behind a young daughter and twenty-one volumes of unpublished, pathetic poetry."

This made me realize that I wanted to write, but also that I wanted to really LIVE. I started to remember childhood dreams I had harbored. Oh yes! I want to be an artist! I want to travel the world! I want to write romances and fairy tales! I want to be a princess! I want to be a cowgirl! I want to be that crazy lady who lives at the end of the lane and has magic gardens and forty cats! I had to resolve those fantasies with who I had become—a marketing executive wearing cheap pantyhose and badly fitting suits, speaking at conferences where I didn't want to be, managing problems that would never, ever be solved.

To get in touch with those dreams, I thought back to when I was truly happy as an adult. It was when Maya and I had gone to Paris. I was almost thirty. Maya was nine. I had put off my European adventures when she was born, so I decided, "We are going to Paris!" It was divine. We stayed in the Left Bank hotel where Oscar Wilde died. We ate in all the famous cafes. We figured out the Metro. We shopped. We went to all the museums. We even worked up enough courage to take the train to Giverny and spend a fabulous day among Monet's flowers and paintings. We took a boat ride on the Seine. We ate croissants and drank coffee and hot chocolate in bed. I wanted more of that in my life.

And so I made my list. I want to write books. I want to swim with dolphins (done!). I want to learn to ride a horse (in process!). I want to ride a camel in the Sahara (still to do). I want to go to India when the kids are grown and not know if I am ever coming back. I want to get to know interesting people. I want to launch a magazine (done!). I want to change the world for the better (trying). I want to LIVE!

Later, when I was looking through some childhood papers for clues to my true identity, I found an interesting checklist, a second-grade quiz asking what we wanted to be when we grew up. The boy list had the following things: fireman, policeman, cowboy, astronaut, soldier, baseball player. The girl list was: mother, nurse, school teacher, airline hostess, model, secretary. I had checked off mother and teacher, and penciled in at the bottom "art teacher."

But according to my parents, I had to be "in the family business." In retrospect, their expectation was probably a good thing because it pushed me into business, which I probably wouldn't have gone into otherwise. I finally decided that to stay in the family business, I was going to make my job into something I really enjoyed. Then, I started to love what I was doing.

Some people would say this was when the trouble all began. I would say this is when the pleasure was born. Finding my pleasure was a difficult birth. But like all births, it was so worth it.

THINGS TO DO IN LIFE—MAYA

I love making lists. So now I'm going to make one of all the things I would love to do in my life, in no particular order:

- Be a published author, write a best seller or two.
- Write a screenplay. Be in a movie. Write songs, record them, and release them. I never want to stop being creative.
- Get married and have fireworks at my wedding.
- Have healthy babies.
- Have a beautiful apartment in a favorite city and a house in the country. They will be models of cleanliness and organization, with chandeliers in every room and matching furniture.
- Have a puppy. My little lap dog, Penelope, will love me in a way nothing else will. She will sit next to me on the couch as I have my morning coffee while reading the newspaper. She will scamper along after me wherever I go, and I will always care for her.
- Design, make, and wear pretty dresses. Which means I'll have to learn to sew.
- Have lots of long, delicious, leisurely meals and conversations with good friends.
- Fall in love.
- Take long naps after an early morning of writing.
- Play lots of games of solitaire with my family. We invented a way to play with as many as eight people, and it is fast-paced and hilarious. And I usually win.

- Rent a house in the Mediterranean and sit around and write and cook fabulous food from ingredients that I bought fresh that morning from the local market.
- Travel all around the world; Go camping in the desert (Miss Maya, Girl Adventuress).
- Be an old lady in Paris who walks really slowly in the middle of the sidewalk and doesn't give a damn about all the other people rushing around, because she was once young and rushed through the streets of New York and Paris and other cities, and now, if this old lady wants to walk slowly, she's gonna do it.

DO IT: WRITE YOUR OBITUARY

Get over the morbid part. We all have to die sometime. This is your big chance to script it the way you want it. Obituaries usually cover a few basics:

- Where you grew up, went to school, and worked
- Your survivors
- Special achievements, honors, awards, or volunteer work
- What charities can people send money to

It doesn't have to be long. It also doesn't have to include how you died. Although feel free to decide on the age of your death. This exercise is all about summing up your life in a few paragraphs as it might appear in a local paper and looking at it from that perspective.

How does it make you feel?

LIST: TEN THINGS TO DO BEFORE YOU DIE

If you need help coming up with your own list, we recommend a book called *Write It Down, Make It Happen*, by Henriette Anne Klauser. But here are some ideas to get you thinking.

- Write the brief story of your life
- Travel to the birthplace of your ancestors

- ∞ Have sex outdoors
- ∞ Build something lasting
- ∞ Do a good deed or a dozen anonymously
- ∞ Put together a photo album or scrap book
- ∞ Plant a tree
- ∞ Invent something new
- ∞ Write down your recipes
- ∞ Heal and resolve your relationships

IN HER OWN VOICE: MADONNA

"To be brave is to love someone unconditionally, without expecting anything in return. To just give. That takes courage, because we don't want to fall on our faces or leave ourselves open to hurt."

"I stand for freedom of expression, doing what you believe in, and going after your dreams."

"Poor is the man whose pleasures depend on the permission of another."

PLEASURE REVOLUTIONARY: MADONNA— POP STAR, MOTHER, ACTRESS, WIFE, BUSINESS WOMAN

WHY WE LOVE MADONNA

Maria—The first time I heard Madonna was in an aerobics class. We were doing leg lifts and ab work to "Holiday." It was a catchy tune, disco-like, yet not quite disco. It made me want to . . . do aerobics.

When I finally got my MTV, after months of scrawling on my cable bill "I want my MTV!" I saw the videos for "Lucky Star." I went right out and got the record album. It was vinyl. The drummer in the band I was hanging out with in college pooh-poohed Madonna as a flash-in-the-pan, one-hit wonder.

"Oh no," I said. "She is going to be huge."

Maya—I am convinced that I actually witnessed Madonna's infamous "Like a Virgin" performance on the MTV video music awards. I was boked at it. Didn't really need to.

Yourself" that got to me the most. The
dustrial fantasy-land. That weird suit
and female. She sang with a power and
owing what it's like to be a woman who
't make waves, be quiet—and then just is

the DJ played "Express Yourself," all the
s, and I *jumped* up and screamed and danced
e the beginning—of the world.

e Madonna in concert in Paris. I brought my
I had an extra ticket. I was really sad that my
because it seemed like something we should
tered the stadium, noting on our tickets it said
at they might not have been up front but at
building. But, with each step we took, Mike and
er to the stage. Finally, we arrived at row 24. It
he French, for some unfathomable reason, label
s. I tried not to cry with sheer joy and anticipa-
donna came on stage, played and sang for hours
e greatest thing in the world.

led me from the show—I was still at work in the late
ned to the excitement in her voice, the cheering in
ed with a mixture of joy, sadness that I couldn't be
verence at how special this woman, this moment, was

night Maya had her picture taken in a Metro photo
it up on the color Xerox and have it in my office. When
in and see it, they ask, "who is that *beautiful* young
mile with pride and say, "that's my daughter."
how lucky I am to have a relationship like I have with
s driving my mother to a meeting one day and played
els Like for a Girl." She didn't really notice the song. Or
e tears streaming down my face as I listened.

But ...
video was an Ay...
Madonna wore was bot...
even rage that comes from k...
has been told to be nice, do...
not able to do it anymore.
    At my wedding, when ...
girls—Maya, nieces, cousin...
like it was the end—no, li...

\
sh...
wea...
came...
was st...
Up in N...
    As a ...
and her co...
work scorn...
that there ha...
but I just wen...

Maya—Once I ...
lyrics started to s...
ing, but I learned a ...
in "Express Yoursel...
dawned on me what ...
loved it all the more ...
years after it came out, ...
to it, but the lyrics don't ...
after school, still watching ...
Nature" said it was OK to s...
Knowing that I could express ...
myself through drugs, misbeha...

Maria—As I grew, so did Mad...
Patchouli that was embedded in th...
    When she went into her sex ph...
sex. I bought the *Sex* book for Lou. ...

Maya—I got tickets to s...
new friend, Mike, since ...
mom couldn't be there ...
share. So Mike and I e...
"row 24." We joked ...
least they were in the ...
I were closer and clo...
was the front row. T...
their rows backwar...
tion. And then Ma...
and hours. It was t...

Maria—Maya cal...
afternoon. I liste...
the hall, and cr...
with her, and re...
in our lives.
    Later that ...
booth. I blew ...
people come ...
woman?" I s...
    I know ...
Maya. I w...
"What I...
that t...

Maya—My absolute favorite Madonna song is "What It Feels Like for a Girl." Madonna knows what it feels like for a girl, and has the ability to express it; she knows what it feels like for a girl, and how it can be transformed; she knows what it feels like for a girl, and she knows that it's okay to be a girl.

Maria—Like a romance heroine, she married a kilt-wearing Scottish lad in a castle in the highlands. Like her namesake, the Madonna, she had a child out of wedlock—like a "virgin born." She's explored different religions, different styles, different faiths and decided that change is good. She has fearlessly grown and evolved. I would like to ask her if she realizes that the woman from the Bible she has changed her name to—Esther—was a mythical woman from Goddess-worshiping times? What she may be searching for is right in her original name.

This past summer we all saw her together, finally—Maya, Lou, and I. Her show seems part canned, part Broadway show, and part religious experience, but I can't help but feel she is amazing. For twenty years, I have lived my life to her music. I have evolved as she has evolved. Her constant edginess has been a model for me. I can grow up without growing "old." I can be a powerful woman and still feel sexy, delight in fashion, and not be held back by anything.

During Madonna's "Music" tour, Maya bought me the cowboy hat from her web site. I tore off the tacky chain around the brim and wear it plain. It's black felt, perfectly formed, and looks right on my head. I wear it to our land where we are building a house (and I feel like Barbara Stanwyck in *Big Valley*, saying "This is MY land"). I wear it when I go to riding lessons, listening to country music. I wear it when I most feel like me, but I have Madonna to thank for it. I have Madonna to thank for a lot of things.

⁓

CHAPTER 10

Open Yourself Up
to the Universe

*Pleasure will give
you signs if you choose to look*

PRAYER TO THE UNIVERSE—MARIA

Right before I met my husband I sent out a prayer to the universe. I made a list of all the things I was looking for: honesty, a sense of humor, someone who would be there for me. When I met him shortly thereafter, I made a mental note. Prayers to the universe work. I was really, really ready, too. I had given up all my preconceived notions of what my soul mate would look like, act like, and be like. I put total faith in the universe to bring me what I *needed*, not what I thought I wanted. More than I could have ever imagined, Lou is what I need. And I probably wouldn't have recognized him before I was ready to.

But let me tell you about Angela, a hospice nurse—a truly angelic, sweet, beautiful woman—who spends each day helping people to die. I met her at a spa when her father brought her along to a company meeting we were having. At thirty, she was clearly in need of some rest and care, and was also ready for finding her true love. She was at that magic place where need and total surrender to the universe combine.

Right before I left I sat with her in front of a cozy fire and told her about my story. I told her she could do it too, but the secret is to be truly open to what the universe sends in answer. It may not be who or what she expected, but it would be right for her.

A few weeks later I got a very excited call from her father. As soon as I heard his voice, I knew what he was going to tell me. He had dragged Angela with him on a cruise to Antarctica. Lo and behold, she fell madly in love with a scientist on board and he had fallen madly in love with her.

"Whatever you said worked!" he said to me.

A few months later when I ran into her dad at another meeting, he informed me that they were now engaged.

Lots of women who are desperate to find a man are looking for all the wrong things. They are looking for a man the same way they look for a piece of jewelry. They want someone who will bring glitter and shine to their status in the world. They don't seem to feel worthy enough to glitter and shine themselves, so they seek a man who is a mirror of what in their hearts they secretly long to be—a celebrity, a high-powered executive, an artist.

Before you find the right guy—it's been said a thousand times but it's true—you have to find yourself. Become the person who you truly want to be whether or not you find a partner. Uncover the essence of your purpose and your soul. Finding your true self, developing and balancing the male and female aspects within you is your own personal sacred marriage. The universe will answer your prayer, when it knows that you are ready to recognize love in all its naked glory, flaws and all.

PRAYER FOR PENELOPE—MAYA

Penelope is the dog I don't have. Yet. She is the one I have wanted for as long as I can remember. She is my mostly companion, my side-kick, my source of unconditional love. I will call her Penelope after Odysseus's wife as a symbol of home. Or she will be, once I find her. Once when I was sad that I hadn't found her, my mom said to have faith and take my own advice—ask the universe. This is my prayer for Penelope. I am asking the universe to bring her to me, or me to her, but just to bring us together.

I have always loved dogs, but the desire really set in about a year ago. I was stopping in the pet store, as I usually do, admiring the doggies in the window and asking to hold one. And deposited into my hand was this little ball of fluff that weighed about three pounds. It was a teacup Chihuahua, the cutest dog I ever did see. And it cost two thousand dollars, which I figured was about six hundred dollars per pound. I resolved to look elsewhere for my puppy.

That night I went home and made a list: "Ten reasons why Maya can and should have a puppy" in order to convince my mom to let me do it. As I read it to her over the phone she said, "Maya, you are twenty-one years old and live on your own. You don't need my permission to get a dog."

I long for the changes that a dog will bring to my life: taking walks, and not staying out too late because there is something at home waiting for me. I want to care for something. I want a distraction from the long hours alone in my apartment. I want a dog so much that cleaning up after one on the street every day seems like a small price to pay. My friends say that what I actually want is a baby, and they may be right, but I think a puppy is a better option for me at this time.

Finally, my Penelope was born on October 6th. She is not a Chihuahua, but a Shiba Inu, which is a Japanese breed that looks like a little fox. I decided to look for a hardier breed. I want a dog that will have the ability to protect me, and won't die if I should accidentally step on it. In exactly five weeks, if all goes well, I will wake up to puppy kisses and offer a prayer of thanks to the universe.

DO IT: ASK FOR SOMETHING, SHOW YOUR GRATITUDE, AND BE OPEN TO THE ANSWER

It's easy, really. Praying to the universe is done in three simple steps.

First: Think about what you really want. Visualize it. Fill your heart with love around it. Don't ever ask for anything mean or hurtful to anyone. It's got to be something positive for all involved. Believe in it.

Second: Feel gratitude to the universe. Express your thanks before you ask or receive anything, just because you are alive and the universe is beautiful and good.

Third: Listen and look for your answer. It's not always what you ask for, and it's not always what you wanted—but the universe responds with an intelligence that is greater than your own.

LIST: THE BEST WAYS TO TALK TO THE UNIVERSE

Write it down. That way you'll have evidence and a record of what you really asked for.

Think it before you go to sleep. Think of it like a bedtime prayer in which you thank the universe and ask for its blessing and protection.

Visualize it. Draw pictures in your head. Cut out pictures and assemble a collage. Or draw what you want.

Feel it in your heart. The universe responds with the energy with which you send it. If you send love, you get love. If you send anger and bitterness, you get anger and bitterness right back at you.

Sit on your couch and think really hard about it and then peel yourself off the couch to do what you can to make it happen. Here's the thing. These prayers don't get answered by sitting in a room and waiting for the doorbell to ring. You are basically asking for good weather and clear signposts on the road in the right direction. But you still have to . . .

Buy the ticket. It's like that old story of the lady who keeps praying she will win the lottery, but she never buys the ticket!

IN HER OWN VOICE: MARGARET FULLER

"I accept the universe!"

"A house is no home unless it contain food and fire for the mind as well as for the body."

"I see multitudes of examples of persons of genius, utterly deficient in grace and the power of pleasurable excitement. I wish to combine both."

"Many things have happened since I echoed your farewell laugh. Elizabeth and I have been fully occupied. She has cried a great deal, fainted a good deal and played the harp most of all. . . . I have turned two new leaves in the book of human nature; I have got a new pink bag (beautiful!)"

"When the perfect two embrace,
Male and female, black and white
Soul is justified in space,
Dark made fruitful by the light,
And centered in the diamond Sun,
Time, eternity, are one."

For human beings are not so constituted that they can live without expansion. If they do not get it one way, they must another, or perish.

PLEASURE REVOLUTIONARY: MARGARET FULLER— A TRAGIC LIFE LIVED IN FULL*

Margaret Fuller was the first female magazine editor. Ralph Waldo Emerson hired her to edit *The Dial*. She was the first woman hired as a newspaper journalist. Horace Greeley hired her to write columns for the *New York Tribune*. She was the first female foreign correspondent, covering the Italian revolution of 1849 for the *Tribune*. But she was so much more than all that.

Margaret was the only woman at the core of the Trancendentalist movement. Emerson said of her: "Beside her friendship, all other friendships seem trade, and by the firmness with which she treads her upward path, all mortals are convinced that another road exists than that which their feet know. . . . Inspirer of courage, the secret friend of all nobleness, that patient waiter for the realization of character, forgiver of injuries, gracefully waiving aside folly, and elevating lowness—in her presence all were apprised of their fettered estate and longed for liberation, of ugliness and longed for their beauty; of meanness, and panted for grandeur." Of him she said: "We [think] this friend raised himself

---

* Written on the 154th anniversary of her death, July 19th, 2004.

too early to the perpendicular and did not lie along the ground long enough to hear the secret whispers of our parent life. . . . We could wish he might be thrown by conflicts on the lap of mother earth, to see if he would not rise again with added powers."

Having been highly educated by her father, Margaret was an activist in the educational reform movement. She taught for the educational radical Bronson Alcott (the father of Louisa May Alcott), and believed, "A lesson is as far as possible from being learned by heart when it is said to be, it is only learned by body . . . I wish you to get your lessons by mind . . . think as well as study, and talk as well as recite."

Margaret was a nineteenth century feminist, holding a series of "conversations" with women in Boston to "answer the great questions. What were we born to do? How shall we do it? Which so few ever propose to themselves 'till their best years are gone by.'" Elizabeth Cady Stanton called the meetings "a vindication of women's right to think." Margaret did not believe that women should view themselves as the oppressed victims of a history of patriarchy; she saw the human and spiritual potential for men and women to view themselves as "the two halves of one thought." She believed that "Male and female represent the two sides of the great radical dualism. But, in fact, they are perpetually passing into one another. Fluid hardens into solid, solid rushes to fluid. There is no wholly masculine man, no purely feminine woman."

In 1845 Margaret published *Women in the Nineteenth Century*, rife with references to goddesses and heroines of times past. She "aimed to show that no age was left entirely without a witness of the equality of the sexes in function, duty and hope," but that the general course of history and oppression was not just stunting the growth of women, but of men as well. She wrote that men have "educated woman more as a servant than a daughter, and found himself a king without a queen. The children of this unequal union showed unequal natures, and more and more, men seemed the sons of the hand-maid, rather than princes."

Of her, Edgar Allen Poe wrote, "Humanity is divided into three classes: Men, women and Margaret Fuller."

Going beyond the Trancendentalists and the feminists, she envisioned an androgynous god who would be worshiped with "religious self-dependence." Resolved not to marry unless she could be her true self in a relationship—an ideal she carried deep in her soul—she met, fell in love with and married an Italian marquis many years younger. The real tragedy would have been if she had never known such love. She had gone to Rome as a foreign correspondent, and was swept up into the cause of liberation. At the age of thirty-seven, she bore a son named Angelo. Although her husband was not well educated, she wrote, "His love for me has been unswerving and most tender. I have never suffered a pain that he could [not] relieve. . . . In him I have found a home, and one that interferes with no tie."

After the revolution failed and all her husband's family support and finances were lost, the couple knew they had to return to the United States and reluctantly boarded a ship back in 1850. Within sight of the shore of New York, a terrible storm arose and the ship was sunk. Survivors said she refused to swim to shore and be separated from her family. She spent the time singing to her son, Angelino.

Create the World Around You

WHAT IF YOU DISCOVERED YOU HAD A MAGIC WAND THAT you could wave and fill your life with pleasure? Athletes, artists, inventors, and writers all know that pleasure starts in your head. And you do have such a magic wand—your power to visualize the life you desire and to conjure pleasure.

After you have uncovered who you are and what you truly desire, you can learn how to direct your energy to create more pleasure in your work and the world around you, with your family and your partner. We hope that this section will help show you how.

But remember: What goes around, comes around. The law of karma dictates that if you choose to conjure in ways that give you pleasure but harm or hurt others, you will ultimately also hurt yourself. If you conjure the forces of love, the love that will return to you feels limitless. Sometimes, your choices will not be black and white. You may have to decide to do something that does cause some hurt feelings to others but is necessary for you, or for "the greater good" of your family, or business, or neighborhood. If you make these tough changes with love, however, even those who feel hurt usually end up better off. Those decisions take deep courage, and the universe rewards them.

The road to pleasure is not always smooth and easy. Sometimes there are skirmishes and traffic jams along the way. But if you pack your toiletry kit of little pleasures (lipstick, some good music, and a comforting snack), you'll be sure to enjoy the journey.

THE SECOND FACE OF THE GODDESS

The Mother

From being a virgin (she who is one unto herself), the Goddess transforms, through the pleasure of sex, into a mother. We see the Goddess most often in the image of the Madonna. The familiar sight of Mary and the baby Jesus can be traced back to the ancient Egyptian equivalent: the Goddess Isis and her son/consort Horus—the ancient power of yo' mama.

An archetypal mother, she holds the power of creation in her body and blood (the ancients believed babies somehow came from menstrual blood). She provides unconditional love, compassion, and devotion. She is always there for you—at night when you are frightened or sick and during the day when she supports you and your accomplishments. No matter what your relationship with your own birth mother, this universal Great Mother figure is with you always—encouraging you on your journey to tap into your own power of creation and love.

CHAPTER 11

Eat Alone in Restaurants

Pleasure can be served on a plate

TO SERVE OR BE SERVED: WHY SOMETHING SO SIMPLE IS SUCH A POWERFUL FIRST STEP—MARIA

I love food. I get far too hungry to give up a meal just because I don't have anyone to share it with—or to settle for takeout fast food because I'm too frightened to go into a restaurant alone. A woman needs her nourishment.

The first time I ate alone in a restaurant I was also traveling alone and ate in the hotel restaurant, which wasn't too awkward. But the second night I went to a fancy local restaurant in Santa Fe, New Mexico, where part of the appeal was food that you just couldn't get in Pennsylvania. People stared at me as I walked in. I didn't know if it was because I was alone or because I looked twelve (I was twenty-one). After a few minutes, people got back to their own dinners and I got on to mine.

Since then, I have eaten alone in restaurants hundreds of times, sometimes just because I feel like it. I get my share of room service, but there is no substitute for getting out of a hotel room, seeing where you are, and tasting the local food while watching the local people. To this day, though, I still have to fight that awkward, stomach-wrenching moment when I first walk in the door alone. Why is that so hard? Why do so few women still to this day go out to eat alone? I've thought about it a lot (while dining alone) and have come up with four theories:

Theory #1: Most women have been brought up to serve rather than be served. We are really good at making dinner, clearing the table, doing dishes. But it's hard to just sit there and not say to the people bussing the tables, "Here, let me help you with that." As it is, I end up giving them lots of sympathetic smiles.

Theory #2: Until about twenty years ago, restaurants were men's domain. Women were perfectly capable of getting dinner on the table at home, but people believed all the great chefs were men. Even Julia Child didn't have her own restaurant, and many of the finest restaurants catered to businessmen as clientele.

Theory #3: Until fifty years ago or so, it wasn't socially acceptable for women to go anywhere alone; they had to be chaperoned. Once they were married, they had to be with their husbands or lady friends. A woman dining alone would have been seen by others as having loose morals, and not caring about her "reputation." God forbid.

Theory #4: It's only in the last twenty years or so that women began earning enough money to pay for a dinner—without needing to get permission or feel guilty for using it to enjoy being out alone. When I was younger I always was thrilled when my father would take Maya and me out to dinner. He loved a good restaurant and we loved getting a free meal. I even invented the "Restaurant Rules" for her so she would behave well enough that he would keep inviting us out. (No running. You don't have to eat it but don't make a fuss about it. No loud talking or crying.) But I also remember the pride I felt when I could finally reciprocate and pay for *his* meal. Now I can afford to go to any restaurant I want. Sometimes I take family or friends. Sometimes I go alone.

We women have thousands of years of conditioning and residual fear to overcome every time we walk into a restaurant alone, sit down and enjoy being served, and eat a delicious meal that we didn't have to cook. No wonder it seems so daunting. Who knew that my hunger for good food was such a radical step? I didn't back when I first went to that Santa Fe restaurant. Here I thought I was just going out for a good meal.

Check please!

WRITING IN RESTAURANTS—MAYA

I have a waiter fetish. There is just something about a man attending to my every whim with a smile. Though I have known waiters in other situations, I only find them sexy at work, which means I need to spend a lot of time in restaurants.

I go alone. At first I did it because none of my friends cared to spend the money. Now I do it because it became my favorite thing. I love to go in the afternoon, when restaurants aren't as busy. I bring a pen and some paper, order a drink and some food, and settle in. I speak to no one except the waiter and the invisible audience I am writing for.

Like most of my habits, I practiced them in my head before I ever performed them in real life. I was a writer in a café long before I was old enough to go out alone. I owe that vision to Hemingway, particularly the first story in *A Moveable Feast*, "A Good Café on the Saint Michel." In it, he is writing a story in Paris about a place in Michigan. Hemingway probably actually wrote the story in Cuba, but the geographical place is irrelevant, because all you are aware of, like the writer in the story, is the café setting, the drinks he orders, the rearrangement of the dishes on the table to make room for more and more pages, and the sheer exercise of writing and scratching pencils on paper. Sometimes he looks up, transfixed by a girl alone at a table not far from his own. Reading that story, over and over, I could never decide if I wanted to be the mysterious girl or the writer. I decided there was no reason I couldn't be both.

One summer, I ended up in Paris, the perfect place to combine my favorite loves—waiters and writing in cafés. The waiters are often gorgeous (and more often absent, leaving a girl to her work) and the coffee is strong. In Paris it is perfectly acceptable, even glamorous, to sit for a few hours alone and write or watch the other people passing by. The language barrier, at least for me, rules out distracting conversations even though a girl alone writing is intriguing to some men, and I've sometimes had to shoo them away.

Moving to New York City really made me a writer. Horrible apartments and roommates watching television incessantly forced me to go out. At first I simply wrote in my journal for hours. As more and more pages got covered in my inky black cursive, I got more and more adventurous in what I wrote. I started in on fiction, short stories and even novels.

One of my favorite authors, Tom Robbins, gives this advice about writer's block—sit in the same place every day and eventually the muse will know where to find you. In college, when I had an assignment due, I walked past the library to a certain café on Avenue A that is always full of people alone, with their laptops and notebooks. I still go there once in a while. Finding a place like that helped my writing and made it seem more acceptable to go out alone.

After years of going to cafés, I made the jump to going to a restaurant alone. I didn't have my props, a pen and paper or even a magazine. But I had hours of practice on being alone behind me, so I sat there alone and enjoyed my lunch. The food was not particularly memorable, but I was and still am proud of myself for sitting through a bowl of chicken soup with quiet thoughts to myself as a side dish.

DO IT: EAT ALONE IN A RESTAURANT

This sounds harder than it is. Feel your fear, embrace it. Now get over it.

Pick your spot. If you can afford it, go somewhere nice where the wait staff are paid to be friendly. We actually love hotel restaurants in big cities, because they are often used to women dining alone. Indulge yourself for once.

If you can't afford it, or you are really afraid, go somewhere cheaper and quicker, where it doesn't matter much . . . a diner, or a chain restaurant. You can work your way up to something more leisurely and luxurious.

This week is a perfect week for you to try it out. If you need an excuse for your husband or kids, tell them you are going out shopping or to a movie. You can even tell them you are meeting a new best friend—you!

LIST: HOW TO GET THROUGH EATING ALONE YOUR FIRST FEW TIMES

Make a reservation. It helps knowing that they are expecting a single woman. And often, even "fully booked" restaurants can make room for a single diner.

If you need to look busy, it's fine. Reading a book or newspaper or writing in a journal are perfectly acceptable pastimes.

Know that you don't have to do anything if you don't want to. You can eavesdrop, fantasize, stare blankly into space, or just watch other people. A restaurant is the perfect place to begin the process of creating your new life. Imagine your story. Who do you want to be when you walk out of the restaurant?

Don't hold back your ordering because you are worried about sitting too long. We've noticed you get remarkably fast service when you are eating alone, so order as much as you want and savor it.

How to occupy your mind. Make up stories about the other people or yourself. Read. Write. Eavesdrop. Pretend you are Ruth Reichl in disguise doing a highly coveted (and feared) restaurant review.

Leave a 20 percent tip. We don't want anyone to still have the stereotype in their head that women aren't good tippers. Plus, 20 percent is a really easy number to figure out (just take 10 percent and double it).

IN HER OWN VOICE: RUTH RIECHL DINES ALONE IN PARIS, FROM *COMFORT ME WITH APPLES*

"Though uninvited, my mother appeared with the first course. 'Is this how you will spend the next ten days?' she inquired. 'Eating absurdly expensive food all by yourself? Trying to impress waiters? Where will the money come from?'

'Be quiet, please,' I said. 'I'm busy. I want to remember every detail of this soup.' I described it for myself, the cream, the truffles, the faintly nutty flavor that could only be sherry.

'He won't call anyway,' she said, meanly, I thought. I ordered a half bottle of Chassagne-Montrachet to go with the terrine de poisson and tried to describe the captain's demeanor as he served it. 'When I came in,' I told my phantom mother, 'he thought to himself, Oh, a woman, she'll have the salad and some plain fish, and he was sorry he had taken the reservation. But I have turned out to be someone who likes to eat, and now he is a happy man.'

'You're not going to order more wine, are you?' she asked with some alarm.

'Try me,' I said, ordering a half bottle of '70 Palmer. Mom looked at the price and was scandalized, but the captain looked at me with serious interest and leaned in to ask how I liked it. I took one sip and thought how there is nothing, really nothing, like great wine. Mom just faded, like the Cheshire cat, as I began to describe the taste of the special lamb raised on the salt marshes of the Landes to myself. And to Colman. I was not lonely."

PLEASURE REVOLUTIONARY:
THE STORY OF RUTH (REICHL)

Ruth Reichl didn't start out trying to transform the food world and the women in it. She followed her stomach, her love and her desire. She followed her pleasure. The product of an eccentric and often dysfunctional upbringing, food became her stability, her source of sanity. She used her love of food first to cook for herself, then to cook for others, and then to write about food. As one of the most influential food critics writing for the *New York Times,* she was famous for dressing in many different disguises and using fake names in order to trick the restaurant staffs into treating her like a normal person so she could get a real view of the service.

With each review, she helped elevate the taste buds of our whole nation. She introduced us to foods from foreign countries. With her friendly voice, she took some of the hoity-toity French pretension out of the restaurant business and opened up new worlds of culinary delights for millions. Now she's the editor of *Gourmet,* and took that venerable, sixty-year-old magazine to win its first National Magazine Award ever (for General Excellence).

Yes, when you dine alone you may hear voices and entertain imaginary guests. But that's no reason not to do it. Who knows where it might lead you and what you might find. Ruth found an amazing career.

It didn't happen overnight and it wasn't easy. But mustering the tiny courage it takes to walk into a restaurant alone is the same sort of courage it takes to live a full life and find your true self in the process.

AN INTERVIEW WITH RUTH REICHL

When you used to wear the disguises and go alone to review a restaurant, did you notice trends in how people treated you differently depending on what your disguise was?
Ruth: Oh, absolutely. So much of how you're treated is about how you present yourself. There's actually one chapter [in her new book, *Garlic and Sapphires*] in which I dress up as Betty. She's actually a woman I found on a bus, and when I got up to give her my seat, she said to me, "Oh, thank you. Most of the time I feel invisible. Nobody ever sees me." That's what I want to be as a restaurant critic. And I followed her and found out who she was—her name was Betty Jones—and I watched her. And when I became Betty Jones, I was invisible.

At one point, I went out with a friend of my mother's, her very elegant friend, who is also an older woman. She was just infuriated by Betty. Because you know, her sense was when you're an older woman, people really want *not* to see you, and you have to force them to see you. And it behooves you to dress well and take care of yourself, and demand good service. So we're in this restaurant and anything is fine with me *[laughter]* and here is this woman, Helen, just giving the waiter hell and demanding, "I want my food right now. I want it hot." *[laughter]* And a lot of it is just *people treat us as we demand to be treated.* So if you go in as a ragged old woman, you're going to get treated like someone who's not going to tip very well and so forth. And if you go in as someone who looks like you know what you're doing, that's how you'll be treated. We really control how we're treated and it's all image and maybe image is stupid, but it is how you're asking the world to deal with you.

So which disguise other than your true self (because everybody wants to please Ruth), did you feel like you got the best treatment?
Ruth: I truly loved being Chloe, who was a blonde. *[laughter]* I found my inner blonde. Chloe was a very elegant blonde and men went nuts for

her. And she had long red fingernails and she was very made up and put together, and she knew how to flirt—something which I've never known.

You just put on a wig and it came out?
Ruth: It came out. I was like, "Oh, my god. Where did this come from?" My voice changed and I actually went out and picked up a man. But Chloe got treated well because she was that blonde woman, that cheerleader, who all chubby, frizzy-haired girls like me wanted to be.

What would you say was one of the biggest reasons that you feel like you were able to do all of the things that you've done in your life?
Ruth: I think that I've discovered the joy of work. To me, there are two things in life that are more important than anything else. One is generosity. I just think it's important to be as generous as you can in every way you can. Because it makes you feel better inside yourself. It just does. The second thing is sometime during my late twenties I discovered that for me, the greatest pleasure was in working as hard as I could and really doing a good job. I just found that self-respect, for me, comes from working really hard. The more successful I've become, the more opportunities there are to do things, the more I get to do. It's a constantly building thing.

How has being a woman who wants to work changed over time for you?
Ruth: Well, I often think that the worst time to be a woman in the entire history of the world was probably my mother's generation. My mother and all her friends were enormously well-educated, very smart, but their purpose in life had been taken away. All the work that women used to do, tending the fields, being a homemaker, didn't work anymore. One time all women had dozens of children, and cooking involved raising the chicken, killing the chicken, plucking the chicken. Putting a chicken dinner on the table was a full day's work. With all these labor saving devices, today, you go to the supermarket, you throw it in the oven, it's five minutes work. So for that generation there was no real purpose for their lives and they were miserable. Women who've had a bad time themselves I think have a very hard time seeing their daughters succeed.

I feel really grateful that, for reasons I can't explain, right about my age was the time half the women I knew were actually raised to think that some man was going to support them—that their job in life was to get married. And half the women weren't. And I fell into the I-never-thought-a-man-was-going-to-support-me [group]. It never occurred to me that I wasn't going to have to work for a living.

Who would you say throughout your life have been your greatest role models?
Ruth: Certainly M.F.K. Fisher was a big role model for me. Alice Waters still is a moral compass. She's an amazing person.

Do you feel guilty about anything?
Ruth: I feel guilty about many things, but not about pleasure. I don't let anybody here [at *Gourmet*] use the term "sinfully rich." When my son was younger I—like all women— felt guilty when I was at work that I wasn't at home; when I was at home I felt guilty that I wasn't working. It's the classic women's thing. But I don't feel guilty about food or sex or the kind of things that so many people tend to feel guilty about.

Were you raised in any religion?
Ruth: My family's Jewish, but we had Christmas; we never went to temple; we ate whatever . . . so, no, not really. In fact, my father was a devout atheist. My father truly hated religion. Passionately hated religion. And felt strongly that it was the root of everything bad in the world and was going to end the world. And nothing has led me to believe that he's wrong. *[laughter]*

So what do you believe in?
Ruth: I firmly believe that the important thing is to be as good as you possibly can. And I think it's just very important for human beings to believe enough in who we are and what our potential is to behave well. And I think it's hard to figure out what the right thing is.

I guess the one other thing that I learned at some point was *that it's the thing that you're afraid of that you have to go towards.* I've never been sorry for doing something that terrified me. I have sleepless nights and long moments of asking, "Why did I do that?" But the older I get the more I know that the more scared I am of something, ultimately the happier I'm going to be that I've done it. You take a deep breath and you just go for it. It seems to me that one of the big things that women have to lose is the fear. I don't think I'm a natural risk taker. Naturally, I'd like to curl up on my bed with the cats and stay there all day. But the rewards come with the risks.

CHAPTER 12

Give Yourself Permission

Pleasure wants you to act on your heart

WHAT'S STOPPING ME?—MARIA

My mother, sisters, brother and I were sitting in the hundredth high-paid consultants meeting griping about the direction in which our company had gone and our frustrating and often contradictory relationships with management. (We were starting to realize that it was almost as if they wanted us to have difficulties amongst ourselves.) We were also starting to lose a frightening amount of money.

"So," in a moment of quiet, our consultant asked, "What's stopping you from making a change?"

I will never forget the moment. In that second it was as if a giant, sleeping machine came to life—wheels cranking slowly at first, steam erupting, whistles first sputtering and then screeching. In that moment we realized collectively that we had been waiting for permission from "Daddy" or some other higher authority to fix it. Problem was, Dad was dead and there was no higher authority. There was no one we needed to get permission from other than ourselves and each other.

That moment was the beginning of a huge amount of work, pain, tears, sorrow, and revolutionary change that totally transformed our personal and professional lives for the better. Our goal was to return our company to its original forward-thinking, progressive publishing tradition, while keeping the parts of our corporate culture that we believed in—such as treating all of our employees and customers with respect.

We all grieved tremendously over the changes that we knew we were going to have to make. We sadly realized that some of the people we had known forever and even loved were no longer leading the company in a direction the family wanted to go in. We had to act decisively—even if it meant causing pain to others. As our changes unfolded, I couldn't help feeling guilty for causing pain to others, even though I knew in my heart and mind that it had to be done. I even consulted an acquaintance, Robert Svoboda, who had written books on karma, who explained to me that causing other people pain may be inevitable in the course of business, but if it is in the greater good for the most people, then it must be done.

When I was younger and working my way up, I used to pride myself on thinking there was no sexism in our business. I was surrounded by women who held a lot of power. I was strong and competent and didn't let anything hold me back, but I was in nonthreatening, lower-level jobs. As I worked my way up the ladder I had a lot of people to whom I looked as mentors—and I felt I had something to prove to them, to my dad, to myself. But I had to recognize my own power and own it. When I finally came face to face with the much talked-about "glass ceiling," I realized it wasn't so much about sexism as it was about the struggle for power. Men fight for power all the time. They fight for power in business, and they fight for it in politics and countries. We see in every political election (the business "elections" are not so visible) a gloves-off, fierce and sweaty fight. Women, traditionally, haven't been willing to do what it takes to win.

Before our "moment" with the consultant, our family had a management team who had been in control and owned the power unchallenged for many, many years. They had had many successes and helped to build the company. When the family wanted to exert more control in order to move beyond our current levels, those managers didn't take kindly to it. The fact that we were almost all women didn't help. One executive quit because he didn't want to work for me. His repeated refrain was, "What do *you* know?" as if I was some sort of entry-level assistant.

I have to tell you, one of the hardest parts of this experience was learning to trust myself, and my own intelligence. It took the help of many outside business school consultants to convince me that I *did* know what I was talking about. I was not about to make such drastic changes to our beloved company without having done the homework. By the time we had decided to make changes, I didn't know where change would lead us, but I was confident it *had* to be made.

So the family took charge and over the next two years the complete management team of more than thirty executives turned over. Some were fired, some retired, and some left by their own choice. We had a major layoff and I went through a massive depression. Going to the local supermarket became a horrible experience, because I would inevitably run into former employees who I had known forever and who blamed me for the loss of their comfortable, happy existence. I got used to being given "the cut direct" (ignored). At one point halfway through it, a dear co-worker actually stopped me in the hall and stated: "This is a revolution." He looked frightened and concerned.

"Yes," I replied. "It is." Unfortunately, even he did not survive it.

We hired a new CEO, Steve Murphy, who had the experience in books and magazines that we needed, plus a true respect for women and our family. Together we saw how cruel people can be when faced with change they don't want. Together, with the rest of the family, we pushed through our desired changes—reorganizing the company around the customer instead of media (books and magazines). Steve brought in an incredible team—the kind of people we had only fantasized about in the old Rodale. The new Rodale was fresh, smart, positive, and happy . . . and our new voice reflected that. Together we agreed that if our mission was to inspire and enable people to improve their lives and the world around them we needed to extend our reach, welcome newcomers, and appeal to a more mainstream audience, while still respecting our long-time, loyal customers.

Was it worth it? Oh, yes, more than I ever could have dreamed. Our business is soaring beyond everyone's expectations. Our family relations are also much improved. Most importantly, we are having *fun*. Work and life are true pleasures.

I often think back to the board meeting before the revolution when I suggested a goal of having a *New York Times* best seller. After all, we publish books and every management seminar I had been to preached the importance of having "stretch goals." Yet the reply was, "We don't do those sorts of books," in a condescending tone of voice. In 2004 we had FOUR, including *The South Beach Diet*, on which, best of all, I lost ten pounds.

We delight in creating excellent books and magazines that help people improve their lives and the world around them. We adore our customers and love to create really exciting new products for them. We even have a very high-level executive, Ben Roter, whose job it is to go around and ask employees, "So, what's stopping you?"

Hint: If he ever asks you, your answer should be, "Nothing!"

MOVING TO MANHATTAN—MAYA

One of the most common conversations among New Yorkers is how we ended up in the greatest city of the world. Hardly any of my friends, or the people I've talked to, were born and raised here. At some point or another, we answered the call, packed our bags, and set off for the city. I'm sure this is not unique to New York. Cities in general have a certain allure, especially for younger people hungry for the options and opportunities that small towns just don't offer.

When I was applying to college, I had wanted to be in New York City. Of all the cities I had been to, this one seemed to fit me the most. Plus, it is a short bus ride away from my family in Pennsylvania. But I didn't send applications to any city schools, because I was told I was too little (four feet eleven and eighty-five pounds) and not tough enough to handle it. In the fall of 2000 I found myself unpacking my bags at a small college in Connecticut. I didn't care for the place, but put up with it for a year. I thought about transferring, but the idea of starting all over and making new friends seemed like an insurmountable obstacle. I went to Paris for the summer, on an NYU program, met some friends based in the city, and reconnected with a friend from high school who was also at NYU. Still unconvinced, that fall I hopped a train for a visit. I met up with another old friend, and had a fabulous time going with him and his friends to a comedy show at one in the morning, instead of the Friday night frat parties. The call of the city was getting louder. Back in Connecticut for my sophomore year, I was horribly depressed. After the freedom of Paris, and all it had to offer as a city—public transportation, museums, shopping, and excitement—and my friends in New York, Connecticut was just too small for me.

And then came September 11th. I had the same first reaction as everyone else, but my second was to ask whether or not I could still make the move. Over the phone, my extraordinarily overprotective mother said unexpectedly, "You have to live your life, Maya." Or die trying, I thought to myself. So I sent in the application to NYU and got accepted. Before I knew it, I was having goodbye parties and packing up my VW until there was barely room for me in it.

I was terrified, and exhausted at the idea of starting over again, scared that maybe I wasn't tough enough. But I was also excited; for the first time, I was living on my terms, or at least starting to. I had figured out what was wrong and how I could probably make it better, and then I did it.

But when my parents were driving me to my new dorm in Chinatown I sat in the back seat, thinking, "I'm supposed to be in Connecticut right now." I had never seen this part of New York before, and frankly it scared me. And I had no choice but to suck it up and pretend everything was just fine. Before I knew it, goodbyes were said, and I unpacked. A soft snow was falling and I was alone. I took a walk. After that, I walked around for hours, for days, discovering my new neighborhoods, restaurants, used bookstores that didn't care if I hung out in there for hours. I went to classes and went out with friends. By the time summer arrived, I had a life I loved that got fuller every day. And I had created that for myself.

Was it hard, and lonely at times? Hell, yeah. Did I regret it for an instant? Nope. And I always get a tingle of pleasure when a friend comes to visit and is impressed with how well I know my way around the subway and the streets. "I don't know how you could live here, Maya," they say. "I don't know how people live anywhere else," is my usual reply. They said I wasn't tough enough, but finally I stopped listening, and gave myself permission to live the life I want.

DO IT: WRITE YOUR MISSION STATEMENT

Every one of us has been given a gift. Your challenge is to discover what your gift is, and then use it to make the world . . . and your world . . . a better place.

Take an hour. Go for a walk in the woods, or the park. Sit on your couch. And ask yourself the following questions:

∞ What do I want my lasting legacy to be?

∞ What will my contribution to the world be?

∞ What is my mission in life?

∞ If I only accomplish one thing, what would it be?

Your answer can be personal, something like "I want to raise healthy happy kids" (which is not so easy!). Or it can be big and more general, like work toward world peace. The key is deciding what your primary purpose and contribution is and breaking it down into a manageable goal. For instance: My mission is to raise healthy and happy children by always treating them with respect and love and feeding them nutritious and balanced meals. That basic goal might just be the most important thing you can do to create world peace. Or you might have a more fun mission: for example—my mission is to bring more laughter into the world. Or, my mission is to create and leave an extremely well-built and decorated house.

Whatever you decide, as long as you truly search your soul, will be right for you. The key is filtering out all the voices you've heard from parents, partners, friends, and kids telling you what *they* think you should do with your life. In the peace and quiet of your own solitude, you can hear your own voice. Trust it.

LIST: TEN GREAT WOMEN WHO HAVE TAKEN A STAND . . . OR A SEAT

Rosa Parks. A black woman, in the segregated South, Rosa Parks one day refused to give up her seat on the bus to some white folks. By listening to her tired feet, she essentially kicked off the civil rights movement in America, showing that taking a seat is really taking a stand.

Margaret Sanger. This trained nurse was troubled by all the unwanted pregnancies and poor health of the women who came to her for help. She wrote a newspaper sex-ed column called "What Every Girl Should Know." It was censored, which convinced her that she had to "bring family planning information to American women." She reviewed different contraceptive devices and provided instruction on how to use them. Obscenity charges forced her to flee to Europe, but she returned, opening the first birth control clinic in America with her sister. When she was arrested some of the clinic's clients loyally followed her along the street with their children in hand. Without her support "the Pill" would not have been invented. More than anything the Pill freed the women of the world to be women first, and mothers only by choice.

Boston Housewives in the Revolutionary War. In 1777 one hundred Boston housewives, outraged at the exorbitant cost of coffee, drove to the warehouse and demanded the keys. When the guard refused, they threw him in a cart. They then took as much coffee as they needed and drove off. Anyone who has ever suffered from a caffeine withdrawal headache should fully understand their actions.

Florence Nightingale. She rejected her parents' plan for her to get married and instead got into nursing, at the time a disorganized, thankless, and dirty business. She made a name for herself in the Crimean War by improving hygiene in war hospitals, reducing the mortality rate from 45 percent to 2 percent. Known as "the lady with the lamp" because of her habit of making rounds each night with one little light, she was also referred to as "the lady with the hammer" after attacking the lock on a storeroom containing nursing supplies she desperately needed.

Amelia Earhart. She was not the first woman to fly an airplane, but she was the one who made it cool. After her first plane ride in 1920, she knew she had to fly. But before she made a career out of it, she went to college, then worked as a nurse and a social worker, while saving up enough money to buy her own airplane. She began to fly full time, setting records, and was the first person to fly solo across the Pacific Ocean. Her final flight was to be around the world. She never made it, but in a letter to her husband (she called their marriage a partnership with "dual control"), she wrote, "I want to do it because I want to do it. Women must try to do things as men have tried. When they fail, their failure must be but a challenge to others."

Harriet Tubman. They called her "The General" since she led Union troops into Confederate territory. An African-American and an escaped slave, she supplied clandestine information as a spy, and led hundreds of slaves to freedom on the Underground Railroad. She committed her life to helping others. Since she was a woman, she didn't qualify for a military pension until her husband, who had also been a soldier, died. When she finally did get some money from the government she opened a home for freed slaves.

Anne Hutchinson. An early Pilgrim with no fear of speaking her mind, Hutchinson offered her own ideas on religion and spirituality: "that the gift of heaven was freely bestowed by God was attained through a direct relationship with the Almighty." She gave talks in her home to both women and men, but eventually was brought to trial by local ministers for heresy and sedition, and for behavior the judges said was "not comely for [her] sex." She faced the panel of men by herself, defended herself well with Biblical citations, and began to preach as she did in her living room. She and her family were exiled from Boston, yet some people followed her to the wilderness of Rhode Island.

Hatshepsut. An ancient female pharaoh of Egypt, from 1473 to 1458 B.C., Hatshepsut got her start as regent while the heir was too young to rule. Eventually, she declared herself pharaoh, started dressing like a man, and received blessings from the high priest and other officials. Her rule was prosperous, her most notable accomplishment the temple of Deir el Bahari, overlooking a valley and lined with statues and reliefs of herself. When her son came of age, he apparently destroyed anything even remotely involved with his mother. Yet she is remembered as the only Queen of Egypt; he is remembered as a jealous son.

Penelope. The mythical wife of Odysseus stayed home while he was lost at sea for seventeen years following the Trojan Wars. Remaining true, she promised the numerous suitors that she would weave a tapestry, and when it was finished would choose one of them for her husband. Each day, she wove at her loom, and each evening by candlelight she unwove her work until Odysseus returned.

Joan of Arc. Most of us try not to listen to the voices in our heads, but Joan did, put on some armor, and led soldiers into battle. Under her leadership, the French emerged victorious from a war with England. After that, Joan found she liked wearing men's clothes, particularly pants, which scandalized the boys in charge. Ordered by the court to put on a skirt, she refused and for that, and only that, she was burned at the stake.

These women took a stand and changed history. Their personal sacrifices can inspire you to take a seat or a stand in your own way. You may, or may not, change history, but you will definitely change your life.

IN HER OWN VOICE: KATHERINE GRAHAM

"What got in the way of my doing the kind of job I wanted to do was my insecurity. Partly this arose from my particular experience, but to the extent that it stemmed from the narrow way women's roles were defined, it was a trait shared by most women of my generation. We had been brought up to believe that our roles were to be wives and mothers, educated to think that we were put on earth to make men happy and comfortable and do the same for our children . . .

"Women traditionally also have suffered—and many still do—from an exaggerated desire to please. . . . Although at the time I didn't realize what was happening, I was unable to make a decision that might displease those around me. For years, whatever directive I may have issued ended with the phrase "if it's all right with you." If I thought I'd done anything to make someone unhappy, I'd agonize. The end result of all this was that many of us, by middle age, arrived at the state we were trying most to avoid: we bored our husbands, who had done their fair share in helping reduce us to this condition, and they wandered off to younger, greener pastures."

"What the women's movement eventually did for me personally was to help me sort out my thinking. Most important to me was not the central message of the movement—that women were equal—but that women had a right to choose which life-style suited them. We all had a right to a frame of reference other than that we were put on earth to catch a man, hold him, and please him. Eventually I came to realize that, if women understood this and acted on it, things would be better for men as well as for women."

PLEASURE REVOLUTIONARY: KATHERINE GRAHAM GIVES HERSELF PERMISSION

In her Pulitzer Prize–winning autobiography *Personal History*, Katherine Graham tells a classic story of a young woman filled with brains and fire almost snuffed out by a traditional marriage. Yet after her husband killed himself, she faced up to running the family business, taking it further and higher than anyone else could have.

Kay, as she was known, had an affluent yet somewhat spartan up-bringing. Her Jewish father and strong, bohemian Lutheran mother provided her with every social and educational opportunity available to a girl growing up in an anti-Semitic society. Her father had confidence in her and respect for her. "He somehow conveyed his belief in me without ever articulating it, and that was the single most sustaining thing in my life. That was what saved me," she wrote.

From the moment her father bought the *Washington Post* in 1933, she and her whole family were immersed in the day-to-day running of a paper. Even while she attended Vassar and then transferred to the University of Chicago, they kept in close touch.

After college she worked for *The San Francisco News* and got in-volved in the labor movement there, reveling in her freedom and on-the-job learning. But her father wanted her back at the *Post*, so she returned a year after graduating from college. Up until the time she married Phil Graham, she was treated by her father as his successor. Afterward, her husband, slightly bothered by her wealth, insisted they live off his salary, and that she immerse herself in being a wife and mother. She described her pregnancy to a friend:

"I resigned myself quite contentedly to the life of a vegetable. I went to cooking school in the morning, had lunch with friends, sat in the sun with other pregnant ladies, talked, gossiped, did everything in short that's in the books including laying out my husband's slippers and smoking jacket. (I'm serious I assure you.) And the funniest part of all is that I liked it."

Even though he had no newspaper experience, Phil Graham be-came his father-in-law's right-hand man. Kay had four children and, at her husband's suggestion, wrote a little column to keep her busy and "to make me a little less stupid and domestic than I have been of late." In 1948, fifteen years after the paper had been purchased, it still wasn't profitable, and her father turned the newspaper over to Kay and Phil, though she took little part in running it. In 1957 Phil had a nervous breakdown. For the next few years Kay dealt with the decline of both her parents and the frightening lapse of her husband into manic de-pression and despair. But they both kept busy, helping John F. Kennedy get elected president and helping her daughter with her coming-out party. When Phil killed himself six years after his first breakdown, part of her life ended, and another began.

In 1963, after a period of grieving, Kay was elected president of the Washington Post Company. "Chip Bohlen asked me, 'You are not going to work, are you? You mustn't—you are young and attractive and you'll get remarried.' I said emphatically that I *was* going to work," she wrote. "What I essentially did was to put one foot in front of the other, shut my eyes, and step off the edge. The surprise was that I landed on my feet." Slowly but steadily she observed and learned how to manage a large media business. She also got involved in the world again. In 1966 her friend Truman Capote decided to give a ball "to cheer her up" (the famous "Black and White Ball"). She became a regular at Washington social events, and a renowned hostess herself.

When Kay was made publisher of the *Post* in 1969, she still felt like a pretender because the business world was still "essentially closed to women." She had come to the women's movement slowly, yet she ultimately, at first unwillingly, became a poster girl for the feminist movement.

Kay Graham had almost always been a Washington insider, but when Nixon became president, it was clear he was not on her side. *The New York Times* scooped the *Post* on the Pentagon Papers—a long, thoroughly researched investigation into the not-so-flattering history of the U.S. involvement in Vietnam. But when the government sued and insisted *The New York Times* cease publication, it was Katherine Graham who made the final decision to take a stand on freedom of speech and continue publishing the Pentagon Papers in *The Washington Post*. That decision made the *Post* a player and prepared them all, almost, for Watergate.

In 1972 two staff writers at the *Post*, Carl Bernstein and Bob Woodward, began investigating a strange break-in at the Democratic National Committee headquarters. This inquiry was the start of the Watergate scandal, which would unfold in the pages of the *Post*, thanks to Kay's fearless decision to publish "the Woodsteins'" ongoing reports. President Nixon resigned and the *Washington Post* won a Pulitzer Prize. A movie of the scandal, *All the President's Men*, starred Robert Redford and Dustin Hoffman.

While Watergate was in many ways the pinnacle of Katherine

Graham's career, she remained a force in journalism and Washington for decades. Her long, active evolution into a woman of power and grace is remarkable. She epitomized the integrity of the journalism business and gradually made her family business, with the help of many good people, including her close adviser Warren Buffet, into an enormous financial and critical success. She continued to grow, learn, and enjoy her life right up to the last when she slipped and fell and hit her head after a bridge game with Warren Buffet and Bill Gates.

Kay Graham learned that the only person she really needed permission from was herself.

CHAPTER 13

Disarm Your Dragons

Finding pleasure is not always easy

THE DRAGON IS ME—MARIA

We all have dragons in our lives—events from our pasts that haunt us, difficult relatives, giant fears. My worst dragons tend to be fire-breathing people who I spent a lot of my life fuming about, reacting to, and fighting against. One therapist called these challenging people "my own best enemies." They were teaching me how *not* to behave. Apparently, that was a gift (which I kept trying to give away but kept coming back!).

For example, one boss (a woman) insisted on pointing a finger and scolding ceaselessly whenever anyone (like me) made a silly mistake. She and her boss specifically delighted in humiliating employees in front of each other. From them I learned how to be a better manager. I've also had to deal with others' envy and jealousy, since they seem to come with trying to succeed and be your best. There were always other people who would rather I just stayed small and invisible. From such adversaries, I learned how to be a better person in general: confident in myself and comfortable with other people's success as well as my own.

I wasted many years of suffering getting sucked into other people's pain and dysfunction, believing they were evil dragons I had to "slay" in order to get through a dark force and into my magic kingdom. I fancied myself a girl knight in shining armor, on my epic heroine's journey. Sometimes, I even believed the unpleasantness was all my fault. In retrospect, I *did* have a dark forest to get through. But finally, when I got to the other side I had figured out that I'm a dragon, too. And all of us dragons need healing.

In the beginning I was an injured, cowardly dragon—overreacting to every slight, crawling into my lair to lick my wounds and crying into my dragon juice instead of standing up for myself, or doing something productive. The first time I truly roared and breathed fire was at my father. He was so revered by so many people, including me, but like all highly revered people he was human, and flawed, just like the rest of us. His flaw was that he was occasionally abusive, and could go from saintly to beastly in an instant. After one family dinner at my house when Maya was about five, she and a cousin were acting up. Everything was chaotic (which disturbed my father in general). She and her cousin were annoying each other and she pushed him off the coffee table he was sitting on. My father snapped, picked up Maya and pushed her to the floor, screaming at the top of his lungs for her to go to her room.

In that second I learned to roar. I rushed over, stood between them and in my own fire-breathing voice shouted, "Don't you EVER TOUCH HER LIKE THAT AGAIN!" You could smell the smoke in the air. I was not just standing up for her—mama bear protecting her cub—but was standing up for the little girl inside of me who had often got whacked unexpectedly.

He was stunned, embarrassed. He went home. Maya and I sobbed all night long. He never apologized, but he pretended it had never happened. He never raised a hand again to me or Maya, and treated me with a newfound respect. Far from hurting our relationship, my standing up to him made it stronger. In the few remaining years we had together before he died, I was never afraid again to speak my mind, and he often asked my opinion. Maya and he also became very close. In standing up for myself, and my little daughter, I had learned my true power and a sad truth: Ultimately, his behavior hurt him more than it hurt me. I learned to be a better parent from him, from knowing what not to do and how to manage my own anger more effectively.

I'm still learning, actually—dragon by dragon. As I resolve one relationship another one turns difficult and I have to relearn again how to disarm the situation. (Laying off the dragon juice has helped a lot.) But now I know it's up to me. I can't change other people, but I can change my reaction. And while occasionally the situation calls for breathing fire, and I now know how to do it, my strongest and most effective weapon is the flaming sword of love.

GROWING UP WITHOUT A BIO-DAD—MAYA

I was quite sad to learn, at a very young age, that my mysterious father was not a prince in a far-off land. I would not one day receive a letter in the mail saying I was inheriting a country, and they really needed their long-lost princess back to assume the throne and be queen. With that possibility extinguished, I lost interest in my biological father—for a while, anyway.

I have never met my bio-dad, as we refer to him these days. When I was a kid, the whole absent father thing was not a daily issue for me. My uncles and a grandfather played the part of father very successfully in my opinion. My mom and I were very close. We watched *Murphy Brown* once a week, and I felt a deep personal satisfaction when Murphy became a single mother and told off the nation for thinking there was something wrong with that.

But about once a year after I got a little older, I would have a crying fit over unanswered questions about my "real dad," as I called him then. My mother and I would sit on the couch in the living room and talk about my "biological father." They had broken up amicably, with the understanding that he would steer clear of the two of us. He got a call from the hospital the day I was born, so he knew about me. "He was a poet," she said, "my high school boyfriend." I sniffed, thinking that made sense. I liked to write poetry. At age thirteen, that was enough of a link for me. It was also around that age when I was home alone after school, and the first person to get the mail. When her high-school alumni magazine came, I would go through it page by page, looking for the name of my real dad, and looking for a picture.

When I got to junior high, my uncles weren't around as much, and I realized Lou, my mom's husband, was going to be with us for good. When he would tell me to unload the dishwasher, as he often did, I would simmer inside, thinking, "You're not my real dad." But I was beginning to realize that he was playing the part of father pretty well. He took me to my softball games, taught me to drive, went to my school functions, and had a music collection I liked to borrow from. He came home from work and had dinner with us every day. In high school, when I needed to speak of him to other people, he was "my stepfather of sorts" and my "real dad" was now "bio-dad." It was also around this time that I learned, after another question-and-answer session with my mom, that bio-dad had wanted my mom to have an abortion. Well, I thought, Fine. And that was that.

When I got to college, I was interested in boys and in possibly having a relationship, but I got the idea in my head, probably from stupid classes about Freud, that I could never have a functional relationship because I had never known my biological father. I was affected by a scene in the movie, *East of Eden*, in which James Dean finds out that his mother isn't actually dead, and cries to his father that he has to find her, saying, "I need to know who I am." It struck a nerve. So I cried to my mom over Thanksgiving break, "I need to know who I am." I was eighteen.

When I got home for winter vacation, my mom told me that she had scouted out the situation, and my bio-dad was now expecting an email from me. I had forgotten my desire to have contact with him and was suddenly terrified. What do I *say*? How does one even *begin* to compose that email? I did it, I forgot what I wrote, but soon he and I were exchanging emails on safe topics, like books and music that we liked. It was startling to me how much we had in common in that area—down to a certain two-disk German techno CD, in which we both preferred the first disk to the second. And after only a few emails, he suggested I come to stay at his place in Boston for a night. You can bring a friend, he said. Bio-dad factor aside, I am not a girl who stays in strangers' apartments. I was freaked out and didn't go. And also, as I was beginning to feel, I *did* have a dad. Lou. I still called him by his first name, but in conversation, I now referred to him as "my dad." All of a sudden, the girl who never had a father had two.

I also concluded that the decision that my mom and bio-dad had made years before had nothing to do with my relationships with boys; or, rather, I didn't have to let it be a hindrance. One afternoon, walking from my dorm to the campus center, I said to myself, "Just get over it." I could play the victim and use a situation over which I had no control as an excuse for emotional stagnation, or I could be the cool, smart, and loving girl I wanted to be and knew I could be. Phrasing it that way, the decision became a very easy one.

My bio-dad and I no longer have any contact. I do sometimes have pangs of guilt that I dragged him back into my life only to push him away again. And it's an odd feeling, writing this, knowing that as a book lover he may very well see a book on the shelf written by both his ex-girlfriend and daughter, a book about pleasure, and our life together without him. Maybe he'll look through the table of contents and see this and just have to buy the book (he'd better). I have no bad feelings toward him, or about our situation. He always has been a part of my life even if he hasn't been there in a tangible way. And that's okay.

DO IT: PICK YOUR WORST DRAGON
AND DEAL WITH IT

First, identify the dragon in your life. Is it a person? A situation? A behavior of yours?

Second, commit yourself to resolving it peacefully.

Third, pray for inspiration and healing.

Fourth, do something about it: get therapy, get educated. Take the first step.

One of the most radical things I, Maria, did was to go into counseling with my own mother. Because we worked together, any falling out we had affected all the people with whom we worked. Neither of us changed much, but we get along better and we understand each other more. I have told her that the greatest gift she gave to me was the time and patience to listen—witness—my own experience and allow me to let it out, and then get over it. Sometimes it's worth it to get outside help.

LIST: THE BEST GIRL-POWER MOVIES,
MYTHS, AND FAIRY TALES

Over the years, we have read lots of fairy tales and watched many movies. We have never quite believed in our hearts that fairy tales and happily ever after stories were the passive, dangerous fantasies that critics and sometimes feminists would have us believe. On closer inspection, we discovered that each heroine's secret weapon is love. Now, fortunately, there are lots of new stories made for girls and grown-ups with a positive message. Still, the secret weapon is love. Here is a list of our favorites.

Mulan. Our favorite Disney movie. In ancient China, a young girl disguises herself as a boy and joins the army. She can barely lift a sword at first, but that doesn't stop her from ultimately saving the lives of her lover, the emperor, and China.

Beauty and the Beast. Disney movie, fairy tale, and common romance novel plot, The Beauty is smart and caring, knows when to say no, when to say yes, and how to love. She knows better than to judge a book or a beast by its cover, and through the healing power of her love, he turns into a handsome, heroic prince.

Shrek 1 and 2. Shrek and Fiona discover again and again that looks aren't everything and true love is much more fun than a pretty face.

Ella Enchanted. In this modern fairy tale movie with tons of great cameos, Ella, as a baby, is cursed with obedience—she can't help but do whatever you tell her to do. But she's also spunky and kind and eventually finds that her own mind and will can triumph over a silly little curse. And she gets the prince, of course.

Cinderella. This hard-working girl is tormented by her jealous stepmother and stepsisters. When the prince holds a ball, she seizes the day and draws on help from her fairy godmother and friendships with the animals to go. She discovers that if the shoe fits, she should wear it.

Spirited Away. A modern-day Japanese fairy tale movie that is animated more beautifully than any movie ever before (except maybe *Snow White*). The little girl heroine has to venture into all sorts of magical, dark places to save her parents, who have been turned into pigs.

The Holy Grail Legend. Based on the story of Parsifal and other medieval myths, the Holy Grail is an allegory for the quest for the cup that Jesus drank from at the last supper. Many recent analyses of the stories believe that the quest for the Holy Grail is not just the epic search for a cup, but for the long lost feminine principle in our own lives.

Whale Rider. The Maori culture of New Zealand, like many ancient cultures, has taboos against women and girls becoming leaders. This powerful, contemporary movie shows how one girl overcomes the ancient taboos by following her true nature and appealing to the creatures at the source of their power . . . with love.

Wife of Bath Tale. Written by Chaucer in the fourteenth century, and part of his *Canterbury Tales*, this story asks and answers the question of what women want, hundreds of years before Freud. A young man is on trial for rape. The king wants him killed, but the queen issues a challenge: She will give him one year to find out what women want. The man asks everyone he encounters, and each one offers a different answer, most of them contradictory. On his last day, he encounters a wrinkly, old woman who says she will give him the answer if he will give her whatever she wants in return. They go before the queen, where he gives his answer, "Women want self-same sovereignty." The queen rules that the old woman was right, and the old lady asks for his hand in marriage. They are wed soon after, against his wishes.

On the wedding night, the old woman transforms herself into a beautiful young maiden right before his eyes. She offers him a choice—she can be beautiful at night for his pleasure and ugly during the day; or she can be beautiful during the day so he could impress his friends, and ugly at bedtime. Weary, he replies, "Whatever you wish, dear." And so, because he gives her the right to choose for herself, she decides to stay a beautiful maiden, day and night.

IN HER OWN VOICE: ANN AND BARRY ULANOV, IN
CINDERELLA AND HER SISTERS: ON ENVY AND THE ENVIED

"We need fairy tales at the beginning of our conscious lives, as we need literature later on, to provide us with the essential metaphors of true and false grace, of sin and virtue, of the shadowy textures of our lives and all our ways of covering them up. If Cinderella did not exist, we would have to invent her."

"In contrast to her sisters, Cinderella is ready to meet the prince as a person in his own right, not as a substitute for her own self. . . . Cinderella deals directly with her own reality, and all sides of it, bad and good. She is ready for union with the masculine. She does not use the prince as a detour away from her own self. . . . But he can only find her when she has tried to find herself."

PLEASURE REVOLUTIONARY: CINDERELLA SEIZES THE DAY AND WORKS HER WAY TO THE TOP

Some of our feminist foremothers thought that fairy tales were about helpless, powerless women waiting to be rescued by some prince and that these stories created a learned helplessness in girls and women and false expectations for how our lives would unfold. Some scholars believe, however, that as religion went on its global rampage, eliminating the female-empowering goddess religions, the old stories were cloaked in the innocence of children's stories, hidden right out in the open.

We like to see Cinderella as the story of our journey as women, from seeming powerlessness—or hidden power—to freedom and pleasure—our birthright.

Here is the tale in a nutshell (a tiny walnut shell that fairies sleep in!): Cinderella's real mother dies (symbolizing the goddess buried in our own consciousness). Her father loves her, but he remarries and lets his new wife and her daughters treat Cinderella as a slave (the stepmother represents the new church). But even while she does all the work and gracefully deals with the abuse, envy, and ridicule of her stepmother and stepsisters, she keeps goodness and love in her heart. She makes friends with the animals, with whom she communicates and who help her in her tasks (symbolizing the power nature conveys to those willing to respect it). When the king holds a ball Cinderella really wants to go, but her stepmother forbids it and creates "impossible" tasks to keep her at home (symbolizing the church's barriers to women). After the stepmother and daughters leave, Cinderella appeals to her "fairy godmother" who answers her wishes and casts a spell that will protect her until midnight, clothes her in the finest gowns and gets her to the ball, where she immediately captures the heart of the prince with her beauty and goodness (symbolizing the true appeal and power of the mother goddess). At the stroke of midnight, she runs home, having forgotten her godmother's warning and dropping her glass slipper in her escape. The prince goes in search of her, asking all the women in the kingdom to try on the tiny glass slipper (the foot in the glass slipper symbolizes sexual intercourse and the right "fit" of true love). Only when the prince recognizes that he has not found her in any other woman does Cinderella step forward to show him that the shoe fits her. Their love saves them, and together they rule the kingdom.

In the Grimm version, the fairy godmother is a hazel tree, a symbol of wisdom and knowledge, that Cinderella plants on her mother's grave. Two white doves, symbols of the goddess of love and of the mother goddess, bring her gowns of gold and silver. Cinderella rebels against her stepmother's unjust treatment and goes to the party—alone. This act of leaving the house—we must leave home to find our real self—leads to the happy ending. She follows her own desires, falls in love, and finds her destiny. She doesn't just marry the prince—she *becomes* a princess.

Marriage scenes in fairy tales may represent the sacred marriage, a key ritual in goddess worship that symbolizes the balance and integration of male and female, the power of love and creation that requires both sexes. By integrating our own male and female energies, we achieve wholeness within ourselves and in our relationships. Cinderella and her prince live inside each and every one of us. We all have the potential to anoint them—and ourselves—king and queen.

But Cinderella is also a story about the dangers of envy characterized by the stepmother and sisters. The moral of the story is this: For thousands of years women have slaved away, listening to domineering mothers, husbands, and sisters tell us that "our place" is serving and cleaning up after them. But if we want to free ourselves and go to that ball—it's up to us! And the goddess and her powerful assistants (nature and her many forces) are just waiting to be asked for help.

CHAPTER 14

Live Life by Your Own Rules— Stop Playing the Game

Pleasure rewards the rule breakers

"THE OLYMPIC CHAMPION OF BREAKING THE RULES!"—MARIA

Because I grew up in such an iconoclastic family, I grew up being labeled a rule breaker before I even knew what the rules were. We were hippies before hippies were cool. By the time I learned what the rules were, I had learned something else: the world does not end if you break them.

Some rules, admittedly, are important to follow. Rule "keepers" veer toward safety. "Always wear a helmet when you ride a bike. Don't run on slippery wet surfaces. Don't drive when you're drunk." Other rules worth preserving are those of courtesy—saying please, thank you, and such.

But after that, all bets are off. In fact, it seems to me that there are two different worlds of people separated by a giant chasm. Most people live on the side of the "it's just not done" tribe. In that world little girls try to wear purple outfits with orange shoes and their mums say, "It's just not done!" The message that little girl hears is that doing anything outside of the bounds that her mother sets is not acceptable, and her true self is silenced. That little girl grows up into the sweet woman who says to herself "I really wish I could move to China and open up a shop," but then tells herself, "It's just not done. Can't do it. No one else ever has."

On the other side of the chasm is the land of "no one else." These people feel an irresistible, rebellious pull when they hear people say, "You can't do that . . . No one else ever has! It's just not done!" If it weren't for those rebels, there would be no ships, no airplanes, no computers, no cars, no cathedrals, no cell phones . . . and no bridges across the chasm.

The first major rule I broke was having a child out of wedlock. That was scary. But I also had to trust the little voice inside of me. Basically, I realized that I was the only one who had to live with my decision, so I made it for me instead of others. Since that decision turned out so well for me in so many ways—including making me work super hard so I could support my daughter and send her to college—it gave me confidence to break other rules.

The next big rule I broke was one about how companies should be organized. Rodale was losing its integrity because we managers were fighting amongst ourselves. Before we brought in our new CEO, I brought up, in various meetings and memos, the idea of organizing the company around customer group rather than by product, books or magazines. The responses are, in retrospect, rather funny and endearing. "Your [sic] wrong," wrote one executive. "If it was a good idea, someone else would have done it already and no one has, therefore it is a bad idea," wrote another. Ultimately, I think the managers were more worried about their own turf and jobs than about the customer.

I also learned that ridicule goes with any new idea. It's like a ring of fire you have to walk through. I will take credit for the original idea, but the credit for researching, validating, and executing and then managing our new organizational structure all goes to our CEO, Steve Murphy. Our revenues are up, our profits are up, and we've won awards and recognition that acknowledge the changes we've made.

I expect some ridicule for breaking the rules. After studying my grandfather's life (his biography was subtitled "Apostle of Nonconformity") and studying the lives of other inventive people, I learned that ridicule is a major way that people try to prevent change. Kids on the playground show that they have learned from their parents at an early age that ridicule and teasing keep people from being different or standing out. Once you see ridicule for what it is, it's much easier to live through it. In fact, living through it leads to really cool stuff.

A rule that Maya and I break is: smart, intellectual women don't read romance novels because those books are trash, poorly written, and they perpetuate women being dependent on men to be rescued. In fact, smart women *do* read romances and this stereotype against romances is a form of bigotry against women. Maya and I love them and think they make us stronger, braver, and happier.

To test my hypothesis, I commissioned a major study of romance readers compared to non–romance readers. What we found surprised many people, but not me. Romance readers described themselves as more independent, compassionate, ambitious, and (no surprise) sexy and romantic than non–romance readers.

Because I was raised to not be afraid and because I like hanging out with interesting, different people, I haven't been afraid, generally, to break the rules. So whether it's having a child out of wedlock, reorganizing a company in a way that no one has ever tried before, building a house without a style to call its own, or wearing ancient ten-dollar J. Crew flip-flops to work with my Armani suit, I'm used to people's odd stares and the pinched faces of disapproval. I am reassured that I am usually on the right path when I am ridiculed. I may be breaking the rules, but I'm not breaking any laws.

One of the recent highlights of my life was when our CEO introduced me at a company event as the "Olympic champion of breaking the rules." I was so happy. I always wanted to be an Olympic champion of *something*.

THE UNSUFFERING ARTIST—MAYA

One day in June, a longtime friend and I were on the road to Chicago when I got a call that confirmed that I would be getting a book deal. After years of writing proposals to agents and editors I was going to get money to do what I loved. I was twenty-two and had graduated from college two weeks before. Driving on the highway, somewhere in Ohio, maneuvering stick shift and cell phone, I said to my friend, "Well, it looks like we have a deal."

"But . . . but . . . you didn't even have your graduation party yet!" she wailed. "You have to suffer for three years first!"

"Welcome to the Pleasure Revolution," I said with a smile.

Suffering and being an artist seem to go hand in hand in most people's minds. Images of waif-like people alone in attics feeding off of stale bread and ambition are common. Artists wailing about the torture of being misunderstood, of having to reject friends, food, society for the sake of art! As if novels could only be written on an empty stomach, as if masterpieces could only be composed with frostbitten fingers. My writing class had had long discussions on how students had to give up their social lives to write; one guy cut off all outside influences—books, movies, the radio—lest they influence his mind and taint his "original ideas." Although Flaubert lived with his mother and his imaginary illnesses while writing the great tragedy *Madame Bovary*, and although I, too, went through a phase of courting the muse of bad mood (and ending up with some really bad poetry), if that was art, I didn't want any part of it. Yet, I still wanted to create—particularly to write stories and compose songs.

A few years ago, a friend suggested I cut off all parental support in order to "do the whole starving artist thing." That would be like cutting off a perfectly good arm. Why would I do that? While some see being an artist as cutting off your ear in an absinthe-and-despair induced episode, I subscribe to Virginia Woolf's idea that "One cannot sleep well, work well, live well, if one has not dined well." I refuse to believe that I need to be in the depths of despair to do something I love.

Suffering artists create tales of woe and sorrow, like Flaubert. One student in my writing class showed up every week exhausted, stressed, and overworked, having sat in front of the glare of her computer trying to concoct stories that would make the reader cry in ten to fifteen pages. I thought that was a very unpleasant way to live and work, but I couldn't blame her. Sad stories do tend to grow up to be "the classics."

But romance novelists write happy stories, and some are *quite* successful. This art does not equal suffering, but that doesn't mean it's not art. To write a page-turning, heart-pounding novel is a great achievement. These writers are not starving—for food, finances, or love. They do what they love and people love that they do it. Perhaps suffering artists get critical respect and happy ones get sales. If you could only

have one, which would it be? Or are you like me, who thinks a girl can
have both?

Writing alone in my apartment all day isn't all sunshine, roses,
and well-turned sentences. Sometimes I get lonely, frustrated, or
bored. Sometimes I feel out of the loop when my friends talk about
nine-to-five jobs with benefits, because writing has no set hours—it
calls and you answer. It may not come with health insurance, but it
does have its benefits. I get to sit around in my shorty-nighty all
day. And I get to create, to write and do what I love. That's my
pleasure.

DO IT: COME UP WITH YOUR OWN LIST OF RULES

Think about it, there are rules that you can live by . . . your own rules.
Which are the ones that have worked for you? Or that you have turned
to in your darkest hours? Think about why they have worked. Here are
some of ours:

> ∞ The world will not end if . . . (I don't get this work done
>   or meal fixed or deadline met).
> ∞ Always try to be on time.
> ∞ No sex without love.
> ∞ Always wash your hands before you eat.
> ∞ When in doubt, sleep on it.

So go ahead, come up with your own list of rules. Better yet, pick a
silly one and go out and break it.

LIST: RULES THAT ARE MEANT TO BE BROKEN

Women should be seen and not heard. John Adams once laughed at
his wife Abigail writing to him to "remember the ladies" as he and his
comrades drafted the declaration. The joke's on the guys, though, since
that became one of the most enduring lines of that time. Women continued to speak up and—eventually—joined them in the hallowed halls
of government. If the universe meant for us women to be silent, we
wouldn't have vocal chords. So speak up.

Always put others before yourself. Sometimes, helping yourself *is* helping others. Every airplane safety manual says that you should put on your own oxygen mask before helping others with theirs. We are not advocating unwavering selfishness, but by making sure your own needs are satisfied, you'll have more to give to others.

Don't stand out. Fit in. In other words, stifle your own needs, thoughts, and feelings for the sake of the crowd. Sometimes we want to wear the "right" clothes, read the "right" books, have the "right" ideas, and be in the group. But don't do this because you're afraid of being separated *from* the group. Whether you are in high school or high society, don't fall prey to the "everyone else is doing it, mentality."

Men don't like women smarter than they are. Throughout history, the women who captured the hearts of historical heroes were those who could converse as well as they could kiss. These women spoke multiple languages, had studied history, philosophy, literature, and music. Some were consummate politicians even though they didn't hold a formal office. These women got respect and love. Do not stifle your intelligence for the sake of any man, woman, or friend.

Don't ask questions. Obey. Blind obedience leads to stagnation; daring to ask questions and searching for answers makes life far more interesting. "What if" questions can keep us up all night, but any innovation started because someone wondered if it could be done, and then set about to try it.

If you don't have anything nice to say, don't say anything at all. Sure, some things are better left unsaid, and often being kind, truthful, and polite goes a long way. But this "rule" often is used to shut people up and keep them from saying things that are potentially enlightening but challenge the status quo.

"The Husband and Wife are One, and That One Is The Husband." This lovely idea was voiced by English jurist Sir William Blackstone in the 1700s and used to justify the laws that forbade a woman to own property, get divorced, or have control over her own person. The husband was "lord" and "master." We can only imagine how many women felt trapped by not being able to have "self-same sovereignty." Perhaps instead, the husband and wife can be One, composed of two loving individuals, neither one dominating over the other.

A woman should never ask a man out on a date. This outdated rule just reinforces the stereotype that men chase and women wait by the phone all night. If you want something to happen, often you have to do it yourself. He might say yes; he might have been waiting for you to make the first move. If he says no, at least you tried. If he gets his knickers in a twist about it, you are better off without him.

Rules about when, where, and how to have sex. In the Middle Ages, having sex in any position other than missionary (woman on her back, man on top), was punishable by death. If this rule were still enforced, our population would be reduced dramatically. Instead of abiding by rules such as "never have sex on a first date," "wait until the third date to have sex," and "no sex before marriage," try doing what *you* feel comfortable with. There is no wrong rule as long as you mutually agree.

What fashion says is "in." If you like something and feel comfortable in it, buy it and wear it. Create your own style. If you don't like something, don't wear it just to be trendy. The fashion police don't actually exist.

Keep your hands to yourself. Don't be afraid to show affection. New studies are affirming what we all know in our hearts—friendly, loving affection makes us happy and healthy. Studies have also shown that babies and animals "fail to thrive" if they don't get some good cuddling. This need never goes away, so don't even bother trying to dismiss it. Reach out and touch someone (legally, of course).

IN HER OWN VOICE: VICTORIA WOODHULL ON LOVE

"While others of my sex devoted themselves to a crusade against the laws that shackle the women of the country, I asserted my individual independence; while others prayed for the good time coming, I worked for it; while others argued the equality of woman with man, I proved it by successfully engaging in business; while others sought to show that there was no valid reason why women should be treated, socially and politically, as being inferior to man, I boldly entered the arena of politics and business and exercised the rights I already possessed. I therefore claim the right to speak for the unenfranchised women of the country, and believing as I do that the prejudices which still exist in the popular mind against the women in public life will soon disappear, I now announce myself as a candidate for the presidency."

"I am a very promiscuous free lover. I want the love of you all, promiscuously. It makes no difference who or what you are, old or young, black or white, pagan, Jew or Christian, I want to love you all and be loved by you all, and I mean to have your love. If you will not give it to me now, these young, for whom I plead, will in after years bless Victoria Woodhull for daring to speak for their salvation."

"Man is determined not to give up this domination, and against it I long since declared war—relentless and unceasing war. I desire that woman shall, so far as her support is concerned, be made independent of man, so that all her sexual relations result from other reasons than for maintenance; in a word, shall be wholly and only for love."

PLEASURE REVOLUTIONARY: VICTORIA WOODHULL— FROM FREE LOVE TO TRUE LOVE

VICTORY FOR VICTORIA

Victoria Woodhull was the first woman to run for president. She was also the first female stockbroker, the first female publisher, the most controversial and popular advocate of free love. This woman injected a much-needed spark to the suffrage movement when it was losing its fire. In America in the late 1800s, she scandalized the nation with a life that was in her own words "ahead of its time." She lived life by her own rules, enduring adoration and condemnation, yet she was practically written out of history. We think she should be remembered.

Victoria was born to the resident eccentrics in a small town in Ohio in 1838, the seventh of ten children. Her mother was deeply religious, and talked to spirits; her father was involved in one scheme after another, which usually lost money. Their most profitable scheme was marketing their youngest daughter, Tennessee, as a clairvoyant medium and spiritual healer.

At age fourteen, Victoria married Dr. Canning Woodhull, who had a very limited medical practice and a very extensive drinking problem. With only three years of schooling, Victoria got a crash course in life. She was often home alone, while her husband either drank their money or spent it lavishly on his mistress. She gave birth to a son, Byron, who was mentally retarded, and a daughter who almost died because her husband was drunk as he delivered the baby. At a time when the man was the head of the household, Victoria realized she had to take control if she wanted to survive and she returned to her family and their clairvoyance business. Her father had given her one good piece of advice: "be a good listener." She and her sister Tennessee and the family traveled around America just after the Civil War, listening to the stories of all sorts of people who paid to have their fortune told.

Work telling fortunes gave Victoria a unique understanding of her future audience; while most prominent suffragists preached to the converted upper-class women, Victoria would reach out to unite all women, all men, rich and poor, including the huge spiritualist faction. The stories of other unhappy women trapped by circumstance convinced her of the need for education for girls, rights for women, and free love—meaning that men and women be bound together by love, not laws.

Around this time, Victoria got a divorce and a new husband, a dashing Civil War veteran named Colonel James Harvey Blood, whom she met when she told his fortune. He introduced Victoria to reformist causes. The sisters had gotten rich from their practice and they moved to New York City. From then on, Victoria would live in homes crowded by her entire family, extended relatives, and even her alcoholic ex-husband. Soon after their arrival, the sisters made the acquaintance of Commodore Vanderbilt, who quite liked them, believed in their kind of healing, and had a special fondness for Tennie.

In 1869, the sisters opened the first female brokerage firm, for which Vanderbilt gave financial backing. The press called them "bewitching brokers," and by their own daring and street smarts, the sisters made almost $600,000 in their first few weeks. They moved to a grand house, and made acquaintances with other powerful men of their day.

Also in 1869, Victoria went to Washington, D.C., to attend her first suffrage conference. She wanted to be involved in a big way and the movement needed her energy and her fresh ideas. The women's rights movement at this time was only really concerned with securing the right to vote, lobbying for a sixteenth amendment, but Victoria realized it would take much more to achieve the equality she desired for herself and for other women. One of her reasons in opening her brokerage firm was to earn money and attention for future ventures, and to contribute to the fight for women's rights.

In 1870, Victoria began publishing *Woodhull and Claflin's Weekly*, which a journalist described as "a 16-page paper [that] dealt in finance and fashion, stock jobbing and strong-minded women, sporting . . . , politics and president-making, supporting a woman even for the executive mansions. . . ." It printed stories by the female Georges—Eliot and Sand—and the first English translation of *The Communist Manifesto*. It was more revolutionary than Susan B. Anthony and Elizabeth Cady Stanton's feminist paper, *Revolution*, and more successful. Women wrote to the *Weekly* in enormous numbers.

In 1871 she took the women's movement to Congress, the first woman ever to address them, and she declared that the Constitution's Fourteenth Amendment already gave women the right to vote, quoting, "All persons born or naturalized in the United States, and subject to the jurisdiction thereof, are citizens of the United States. . . . No state shall make or enforce any law which shall abridge the privileges or immunities of citizens." Of this speech, even an anti-suffrage paper, *The Tribune*, offered praise: "All the past efforts of Miss Anthony and Mrs. Stanton sink to insignificance beside the ingenious lobbying of the new leader and her daring declaration."

In 1872 her Equal Rights Party nominated her for the presidency with Frederick Douglass as her running mate. He would have been the first black candidate for vice president, had he accepted the nomination.

Victoria gave lectures that seem the equivalent of rock concerts today, drawing in thousands of people, even in the worst weather, standing room only. Her most popular speech topic was free love: she endorsed monogamous relationships and marriage as long as they were based on love; when love ended, a marriage should also end. She practiced what she preached and caused a scandal.

After a speech she gave in 1872 attacking the capitalist system and referring positively to communism, the public turned against her. A depression hit the country in a few months later, and Victoria's brokerage firm closed. Having raised herself from nothing to riches, she was now broke. Even *The Weekly* temporarily suspended publication, but she revived it for one issue in order to expose the hypocrisy of the most famous, respected preacher of the time, Henry Ward Beecher, which led to the ruin of her own reputation.

The Beecher family was incredibly popular around the country. The Reverend Beecher's sister, Harriet Beecher Stowe, wrote *Uncle Tom's Cabin*. Another sister, Catherine, wrote books in praise of housework and housewives. These two Beecher sisters opposed women's suffrage, Victoria Woodhull, and all she stood for. Their brother Henry had a habit "of taking his mistresses from his congregation" which was common gossip. But when Victoria published a story about his infidelities it resulted in the biggest sex scandal of the time. As a result of that issue of *The Weekly*, on election day 1872, Victoria and her sister Tennie were in jail on obscenity and libel charges. Yet across the country her name was written on ballots. The charges were ridiculous, the trials even more so, yet they ruined her. Her suffragist friends distanced themselves; Susan B. Anthony condemned her. The press was scathing; the two Beecher sisters mocked her in print every chance they got, although brother Henry never charged Victoria for libel, because, after all, everything she had printed was true.

The sisters were in and out of jail for a year but were eventually acquitted and set sail for England, where they turned themselves into respectable ladies. Victoria denied her past, even changed her name to Woodhall. She had divorced Blood, the man who had stood by her for years, under charges of adultery. There, Victoria, the advocate of free love, found true love with Joseph Biddulph Martin, an established, respected banker who supported her unconventional beliefs and was seemingly unfazed by her scandalous past. They lived happily together with her two children for years, until his death. Tennie had married a rich old man and become Lady Cook, but the two sisters, once so close, had become estranged.

When Martin died, Victoria was left with a country estate and a fortune. Because of her devotion and charitable works, the people of the local villages loved her. She died at the age of ninety, in 1927, having outlived all former friends and enemies.

When women finally got the vote in 1920, Victoria was one of the only suffragists who had lived to see it happen. For all that she had done, she was practically absent from the six-volume definitive history of the suffrage movement by Elizabeth Cady Stanton and Susan B. Anthony, appearing only in footnotes. Victoria had spent practically $100,000 (a million in today's dollars) of her own hard earned money to fund the movement. She had risked her reputation to speak out on controversial issues, and she had practiced what she preached—free love, the right of a woman to vote and run for office, the right of a woman to try and succeed in business, the right of a woman to be her own person. Yet for all she said and did, women were her most vicious enemies.

History has proved Victoria right. Getting the vote did not end the quest for women's equality. Women are still closing the gap between what we earn and what men earn, yet a woman today who is successful in business, married to a man she loves, who cares for her children, votes in elections without fear of arrest, and speaks her mind is not at all out of place. We now take for granted Victoria's scandalous idea and practice of no marriage without love. Perhaps now we are on our way into a new, enlightened "Victorian" era—a time when women like Victoria Woodhull are the norm not the exception.

CHAPTER 15

Learn to Say No
(Now That You Have a Voice)

Pleasure is up to you

JUST SAY NO TO SEX, TELEMARKETERS,
AND YOUR KIDS—MARIA

I had a hard time saying no to boys (and sex) when I was younger. I loved being friends with boys. They were interesting and adventurous, but there always seemed to be that point where their friendship turned into lust and I felt really guilty, like it was my fault for "leading them on." Too many times to count I let them have their way with me and felt even worse afterwards, having lost both my self-respect and their friendship. Back then I was a slow learner, probably because I was stoned most of the time. But gradually I learned how to say no.

First, I started saying no to boys and sex. That was quite liberating. It took me a long while to get to that point. Since I learn best by experience, it took a soul-scorching, passionately obsessive, chemically addicting sexual relationship to teach me the full potential of sex. For the first time, I really felt something and when it didn't work out it hurt like hell. It made me realize what I really wanted and needed in a man. I became strong enough to hold out for that.

Then I started practicing saying no on telemarketers. Something about the anonymity was exciting. "No thank you, I'm not interested." Click. Over and over again. I got my speed up to really fast; they barely knew what hit them.

But I really learned to say no when Maya was growing up. She calls me overprotective, which is fine with me. Compared to other parents, I was. But I knew things . . . I knew. I knew what terrible things went on in basements after school. I knew how easy it was to make a wrong decision that you regret forever. I knew how easy it was to find drugs, alcohol, cigarettes. I also knew how hard it is to navigate a life when your parents don't give you enough boundaries, when they are so busy living their own lives that they forget to help you learn how to live yours. I knew how easy it was to tell your parents one thing and do another. I knew how easy it was for a terrible thing to happen in an instant—a car crash or a bicycle accident—that would change your life forever.

Maybe some parents are trying to be cool, or avoid confrontation, but moms and dads seem to have no problem letting their kids stay out late, sleep over anywhere, or drive around with friends piled into small cars blaring loud music. I said "no" to that most of the time. Maya had to be home early. She only slept over if I knew the parents and had cleared it with them—I preferred to have visited their house for an onsite inspection first. She was not allowed to drive with more than one other kid at a time (and no one else until she was seventeen). I knew she could have gotten into trouble at any time. I also knew my strong concern would make her more aware of her actions.

But I picked my battles. She was allowed to die her hair purple in seventh grade (no permanent harm done). When she wanted to pierce her nose, I said she could pierce anything she wanted if she got straight As. When she wanted to go see her favorite band, the Breeders, I was more than happy to drive her and a friend, watch the show, and drive them home. (I was breeding myself at the time—eight months pregnant with Eve.)

I know it's hard to say no and stick with it when a kid will try anything to change your mind: tears, door slamming, the silent treatment. Eve's "killer ap" is a foot-stomping, arms-crossed, tear-stained "plllllleeeeeeaaassssseeee!" I also know they are testing themselves, the boundaries, and me—the strength of my "no." If they easily break through "no," then they don't need to believe anything else I say. I'm willing to be "mean old Mom" when I have to be. It's my job and I do it well. Parenting by saying "no" is a matter of trust and love. Saying "no" is a matter of trust and love for myself, too. It's my fault if I don't care enough about myself to protect my time, my interests, my heart, and my body.

There is something else I know. Once kids leave the nest and go off to college they can do whatever they want. But with a good foundation they can make the right decisions for themselves. And part of that foundation is teaching them that it's OK to say no.

KNOWING WHEN TO LEAVE
THE PARTY—MAYA

At five A.M., I was on a street in New York's East Village, outside of the most disgusting bar in the world. I was drunk, and with two new best friends, forty-year-old punk rockers with whom I was in a band—one without a name, songs, or a rehearsal schedule. In fact, we'd never even been together in a room that didn't have a liquor license. Although I told myself, "You're a rock star!" deep down inside I knew that this band was going nowhere fast, and I would be too, if I kept it up. Taking a taxi back to my apartment in the quiet of an early Sunday morning, I said to myself, "The party is over. It's time to go home."

I faced up to something in me that would say, "I know you're bored now, Maya, but maybe if you hang around for another drink, one more hour, hang on a little longer, try a little harder, things might get interesting." That voice was often a liar, liar, pants on fire. When I listened to it, I ended up feeling bad—from a lack of sleep, or from drinking too much, which then made me unproductive during the few daylight hours I was up.

The "band" had been sapping my creative energy. I spent a lot of time arranging rehearsals that no one went to. I wrote songs that weren't my style, and that didn't really get played anyway. I complained to my girlfriends about my frustration. I thought I was living my dream of being a musician, afraid this was my one shot at my dream of playing in a band. Moving on and saying no seemed equivalent to quitting.

At least that's what I told myself. But after a few more rock-and-roll nights and nonrocking days, I realized I was hanging out at a party that not only wasn't my scene, it wasn't even a party. It was time to call it a night. I realized I was wasting time. So I started to say No.

It was hard, giving that up, until I thought of it a different way. Saying no to one thing was often saying yes to something else. If I said "no" to going out, I was in effect saying "yes" to sleep, to waking up refreshed, to better opportunities. I still go out, but I do not keep the same hours that I used to. I haven't seen five A.M., or that bar, or my punk rocker "bandmates" in a long time. I had fun with them for a while, but things started to change for me. I heard another voice telling me to move on, and I listened to it tell me that saying no to some things was really saying yes to better things.

Soon enough, after that party was over, I met another musician, whose idea of rock and roll was—and here's a shocker—playing music! In a rehearsal studio! Or at his home recording studio! Did we get a record deal? No. Do we still play together? Nope. That party ended too, but I have something more pleasant than a hangover, and something far more lasting: recordings of two songs I wrote, sang, and played guitar for. They may not be hit singles, but they're mine.

DO IT: JUST SAY NO

Come on, you know you want to! You also know what it is you want to say no to. Maybe it's your mother. Or your sister. Or your spouse. Or your kids. Or your boss. Or maybe it's no to that next drink. Next donut. Next debt. Next temper fit. Next pity party.

If you need to practice, do it on telemarketers. I used to be in that business (and sort of still am) and the only reason they keep calling is because enough people keep saying yes. Consider it your favor to humanity.

LIST: THE NICEST WAYS OF SAYING NO WITHOUT LYING

Say "No, thank you" in a polite but firm voice. You do not need to share your reasons. This works best on people who are trying to sell you stuff you don't really want.

If someone invites you to go along with something you don't want to do, try saying, *"I'm sorry, but I already have plans."* You do—not doing it is your plan.

If you have to say no to yourself, try to think of it as saying yes to something else. Saying no to that last drink on a night out seems boring at the time, but quite wise the next morning.

Offer another option. When you offer another option, "no" can often sound like a yes. This is also known as compromising. For instance, in the restaurant reservations office, if a customer asks for something we don't have available, we always offer an alternative. If we're fully booked at eight o'clock, we offer different available times, or the option to just walk in, or the option to call back and check for cancellations.

Have a nonnegotiable "no." Sometimes, if I was invited to something I didn't want to do, but felt like I couldn't say no, my mom would say, "Tell them I said no." *Ninety-nine percent of the time, if a mom says no, it is nonnegotiable.* Once you are grown up, it's hard to use the "my mom said no" excuse. But you can decide what your nonnegotiable no is for yourself. It can be anything that interferes with your obligations to your kids, your Sunday, or your Thursday night TV. It's up to you do decide.

If you find yourself repeatedly saying no, and the person you're talking to won't give in, say, *"I'm sorry you feel that way. Is there anything I can actually help you with?"* Full stop. Never fails.

IN HER OWN VOICE: SOJOURNER TRUTH

"Well, children, where there is so much racket there must be something out of kilter. I think that 'twixt the negroes of the South and the women at the North, all talking about rights, the white men will be in a fix pretty soon.

"That man over there says that women need to be helped into carriages, and lifted over ditches, and to have the best place everywhere. Nobody ever helps me into carriages, or over mud-puddles, or gives me any best place! And ain't I a woman? Look at me! look at my arm. I have ploughed and planted, and gathered into barns, an no man could head me! And ain't I a woman? I could work as much and eat as much as a man—when I could get it—and bear the lash as well! Ain't I a woman? I have borne thirteen children and seen most all sold off to slavery, and when I cried out with my mother's grief, none but Jesus heard me! Ain't I a woman?

"Then they talk about his thing in the head; what's this they call it? [member of audience whispers, "intellect"] that's it, honey. What's that got to do with women's rights or negroes' right? If my cup won't hold but a pint, and yours holds a quart, wouldn't you be mean not to let me have my little half measure full?

"Then that little man in black there, he says women can't have as much rights as men, 'cause Christ wasn't a woman! Where did your Christ come from? Where did your Christ come from? From God and a woman! Man had nothing to do with him.

"If the first woman God ever made was strong enough to turn the world upside down all alone, these women together ought to be able to turn it back, and get it right side up again! And now they is asking to do it, the men better let them."

PLEASURE REVOLUTIONARY: SOJOURNER TRUTH— SAYING NO TO THE STATUS QUO

Sojourner Truth was born a slave, died a freed woman, and was devoted to God, traveling all over the country during her later years, preaching to all who would listen—including church congregations and suffragist meetings. Once she found her voice, she made sure people heard it.

As a young child, she was known as Isabella and watched with her mother as her siblings were sold off to other masters. Her mother told her about God, motioning that He lived in the sky and would help Isabella. As a child she, too, was sold to another master, and eventually freed. All the while she had been talking to God.

As a freed woman, one of the first things she did was track down one of her children, a son who had been sold farther down south, even though that practice of trading slaves had been made illegal. With the help of some strangers, and her persistence in the local courthouses, she finally got her boy back. They traveled north to New York City.

It is unclear how she earned a living there. Her son had some jobs, but more often than not got into trouble. While living in New York,

Isabella came to know a man who called himself Mattias, and followed him to a commune. All the while Isabella had been forming her own ideas of religion, "which involved the traditional solace of a loving God but also added a sense of strength and specialness." Her new spirituality prompted her to rename herself Sojourner Truth, and she set off to preach. According to *America's Women*, she "was the only female ex-slave who pursued a career as a public speaker. Perhaps she was the only American strong enough to overcome the combined insecurities that came with being a woman and being a slave."

What survives of Sojourner Truth's speeches reveals an extremely honest, brave woman. She was often accused of being a man because she dared to speak in public, and had a low voice. But when confronted by this charge in Indiana, when male hecklers demanded that she show her breasts to the women in the audience to prove her sex, she told the men she "had suckled many a white babe, to the exclusion of her own offspring . . . and she quietly asked them, as she disrobed her bosom, if they, too, wished to suck!" Assured in her devotion to God, she spoke up at any opportunity. She had suffered as a slave, and as a freed woman devoted her life to God, preaching the truth that others were afraid to recognize.

CHAPTER 16

The Power of Yes
Pleasure holds you alone responsible for your life

. . . and how he kissed me under the Moorish wall and I thought well as well him as another and then I asked him with my eyes to ask again yes and then he asked me would I yes to say yes my mountain flower and first I put my arms around him yes and drew him down to me so he could feel my breasts all perfume yes and his heart was going like mad and yes I said yes I will Yes.

—JAMES JOYCE, *Ulysses*

MY HALLOWEEN YES—MARIA

By the time I was in my thirties I was much better at saying no than I was at saying yes, especially when it came to social functions. I rationalized that I spent all day in meetings talking to people and managing them and when I got home I just wanted to curl up in bed with a good book. The last thing I wanted to do was go out and see more people and talk to them. Even though I often give speeches to lots of people, I don't like being on center stage. I am really rather shy, and have to force myself to be social. Lou, my dear husband, on the other hand, loves to socialize, which is strange because in general he is very quiet.

But whatever our differences, the fact of the matter is we have lived on Main Street, Emmaus, for all of our marriage and there is one thing that you must do if you live on Main Street, Emmaus . . . you must invite everyone you know to your house for the annual Halloween Parade. We supply food, bathrooms, and hot beverages and our guests get prime seats to our town's biggest night. I have lived on Main Street for twenty-three years and I have had twenty-two parties (I missed one year for some reason).

After ten years of watching the parade, Lou got the crazy idea that we should march in the parade and pull the kids in a wagon. Every fiber in my body said no. With superhuman Halloween strength, I turned the "no" I wanted to say into a "yes" as it came out of my mouth. I said yes for Lou, because I knew it would make him happy. And then Lou told me he wanted to do a '70s theme. I groaned. His '70s are *not* my '70s. It's kind of ironic when you think about it. In Lou's '70s he was a varsity basketball star and straight-A student having the time of his life living the Italian-American dream with John Travolta as his hero. In my '70s I was a smoking, drinking, acid-dropping hippie listening to the Grateful Dead who often was not sure where I was when I woke up. The last thing I wanted was to relive those days. (To this day it astounds me that we married each other. "But we get along," is his answer. It's true. We do.)

So we went to the costume store, where Lou bought a giant black afro wig and a powder blue tux with a ruffled shirt.

"You look exactly like my dead, gay brother." I told him. True.

The only thing I could think of to wear that would totally disguise me was a conehead with Elton John rhinestone glasses. It was truly ugly. I felt very comfortable in it.

On the night of the parade, every guest room was filled with out-of-town participants. The only people invited to the party were those who would march, but a few relatives showed up anyway. We waited for what seemed like hours in the parade lineup between a scout troop and a monster truck "float" of some sort. The disco on our boom box was getting us warmed up and I was thinking this is the stupidest, most unpleasant thing I have ever done and I will never do it again.

When we started to "march," Lou began taking pictures of people lining the streets with a Polaroid camera and handing them over. He started dancing and high-kicking like I'd never seen him before and I thought he truly *had* channeled the spirit of my brother. He was having them. Finally, I called my friend's mom in New Jersey. "Oh, hi," she said. "Brown University is on spring break right now and he's in Oregon visiting his girlfriend." This is why most people call ahead when they want to visit someone.

At this point, we could probably have driven back to school before anyone noticed we were gone. Instead we went shopping. Lia bought a box of hair-dye, and now we just needed a place to do it. She had a friend at Tufts University, so we decided to go to Boston. We called a friend back at school and left a message saying "Hi, we're driving around New England and don't know when we'll be back." We had now been awake for twenty-four hours, and I was getting funny looks for the cowboy hat I was still wearing.

After getting lost in Boston and the surrounding area for a few hours, we arrived at Tufts, finding Lia's friend cleaning up from a sorority party the night before. We stayed for about forty-five minutes, just long enough to dye Lia's hair in the bathroom sink of a dorm-room bathroom, and got back in the car for the long drive home. We sang along to a CD that skipped on most of the tracks, we listened to the radio, and we never ran out of things to talk about. I can't remember a single thing we discussed, but I started to lose my voice by the end of the trip.

And finally, after being awake for over thirty hours, we walked into our hall, still wearing the same clothes, the cowboy hat. With hoarse voices, we recounted the story of our spontaneous adventure.

It's amazing where saying, "What the heck, yes, let's do it," will lead you. We thought we were just going out for French fries, and we ended up with a road trip that sealed our friendship. That trip was one of my first big, strong tastes of freedom. It gave us the magical feeling of saying yes and seeing where the mood would take us. And to think we might have just gone home and gone to bed.

DO IT: JUST SAY YES

You've been hankering to say yes to something deep down in the secret velvet of your heart, something you have been pining for. Think of the happiness you'll have when it's all said and done.

The trick is to catch yourself the next time you're about to say no automatically, without thinking, just out of habit—even if it's to yourself.

a blast. I started to see people I knew. They were laughing and poin
ing. And suddenly I realized, they didn't recognize me! So I starte
shaking my butt and dancing just a little.

By the time we got to the triangle, the main stage of the parade
where the TV cameras and judges are, the kids were all asleep in their
wagon and I was dancing in public like I hadn't since . . . well, the '70s!
That was not bad at all.

We crossed the finish line and discovered that we had won third
place for a "non-float" group (seventy-five bucks!). It felt like we had
just won the National Championship of Disco. We were all extremely
proud. I had survived and my husband was totally in his element.

Ever since then if I get the urge to say no to someone's crazy idea I
think back to my night as a conehead, dancing anonymously on the
streets of my home town. And I say yes!

SURE, WHY NOT?—MAYA

It was a Friday night during my freshman year of college, and I had
come back to my dorm at about three A.M., and run into my friend
Lia in the hallway. "I'm hungry," she said, "let's go to the diner." I put
on a black-and-white cowboy hat, and we got in the car. Lia did the
driving, since she hadn't been drinking.

At the twenty-four-hour diner, we were just talking, eating French
fries. At about four-thirty we realized the sun was going to come up
soon and it would be cool to drive to the beach and watch the sunrise.
We set off, but soon saw signs for Providence, Rhode Island. Lia and I
just looked at each other and nodded. We weren't going to the beach
anymore, we were going to Providence, where we both had friends at
Brown University who we wanted to drop in on. After we agreed, we
pulled over to fill up the tank. Lia bought a pack of cigarettes and some
Diet Cokes: she constantly has a cigarette in one hand and a Diet Coke
in the other. We also bought a disposable camera to document our
spontaneous road trip. I still had on the cowboy hat.

At seven in the morning we pulled into Providence. At this point
we had both been awake for almost twenty-three hours. It was too
early to call anyone, so we just wandered around. From about nine to
eleven in the morning we tried to track down our friends. We used
campus phones, directory assistance, the phone book, but couldn't find

When you feel that no coming on, check it out. Turn it around a bit on your tongue. See if that no really, deep down, would rather be a yes. If it does want to change, just say yes.

LIST: THINGS TO WHICH WE USUALLY SAY NO, BUT SHOULD SAY YES

Say yes to trying new things. Go somewhere you've read about, or walked by but never entered. Wander. When you go shopping, try on something you would probably never wear or buy, just for kicks.

Say yes to acting "out of character." "Oh, I don't do that," you may say, even if you really want to do it. Dancing, for example. No one is stopping your reinvention of yourself except for you.

Say yes to making a sexual fantasy real. We strongly encourage you do this with a partner with whom you feel comfortable. And, unless you're trying to get pregnant, use protection. But that should be the only limit on your imagination.

Say yes to taking a day off just for you. Don't wait to get sick to take a day to lounge around in bed, read magazines, or go for long walks in the woods. Skip the errands, the shopping, the work and enjoy your freedom, and your health, if only for a day.

Say yes to yourself. Anytime we berate ourselves with inner talk like, "I'm not good enough," "I don't deserve it," or "I couldn't possibly" we burn bridges of potential pleasure. You *are* good enough. You *do* deserve it. And you *could* possibly do whatever you desire.

IN HER OWN VOICE: ALICE WATERS

"People have always foraged during the seasons for what was close by. They picked it, and they brought it to the marketplaces, and they sold it to people in the neighborhood. People brought it home, cooked it, and ate it with their families. It's ritual—sacred ritual, I think, in most households around the world."

"These kids at the school, they're hungry, they want to eat; but they're also hungry for attention. They're hungry for everything that comes with that food. That's what they're really hungry for: somebody to sit down and talk with them."

"Organic produce is pure and wholesome and delicious and alive when I get it. And nine times out of 10, it's picked very ripe. . . . Yes, it takes a little longer to shop at the farmers market, but what you get, in my mind, is an experience that enriches one's life. It's an experience of connecting with people. It smells good. It tastes good. It has a good feeling about it. There's no way that that kind of experience can't seduce people."

"All who offer sacred hospitality are rewarded in the very same way: Our dwellings become as temples and our branches intertwine."

PLEASURE REVOLUTIONARY: ALICE WATERS— GODDESS OF GOOD FOOD

Alice Waters changed how Americans enjoy food forever. Back in the 1970s when she opened her little restaurant called Chez Panisse in Berkeley, California, there were two kinds of food in America: bad-tasting but healthy and good-tasting but unhealthy.

Alice, a Jersey girl, had gone to France, where she experienced an "awakening" of what food and eating could be—fresh, local, seasonal, social, alive, and filled with pleasure. From that experience, she had the radical idea that organic, seasonal, and fresh food *tasted* better (health effects being a bonus), and translated her belief into incredible, delicious, gourmet food.

Back then (imagine!), she had trouble finding good, fresh food in California, so she drove down to the docks. She hauled herself out to the farms. She found people who could make real bread. Slowly, gradually, she became both the mother of modern American cooking and the "patron saint for small organic farmers." Because the food at Chez Panisse was so delicious and pleasurable, her invention spread across the country (and even back to France). Her passion for fresh, delicious food has done more to improve how Americans eat than almost anything we can think of.

But she's not done yet. Now, her mission is to take her food revolution into the public schools of Berkeley, teaching the kids how to grow, cook, and eat good food. The Chez Panisse Foundation will be developing curricula, renovating kitchens and cafeterias, planting gardens, and studying how eating well and the responsibility that growing and cooking food inspires affects behavior, attendance, and test scores.

We held this interview over dinner at Chez Panisse, where every night there is one menu for everyone—like going to a fabulous dinner party where each course is a delightful surprise. And Alice reigns supreme.

INTERVIEW WITH ALICE WATERS—COME TO YOUR SENSES

What gives you the most pleasure?
Alice: Making other people feel really good about something. Making them comfortable. Giving them some kind of experience that is pleasurable. That's very satisfying to me.

Where do you think that desire comes from?
Alice: I guess a little bit from my having had that experience myself of going to France, when I was nineteen, at that impressionable age, and having people serving me delicious food. I was changed by that. And it made me think that I could give people that experience that they'd never had before. The experience changed me and the course of my life.

You were twenty-seven when you started Chez Panisse. What made you as a woman at the time feel like it was possible?
Alice: It's very hard to say. I feel like I had an awakening, a sort of sensual awakening. I felt things for the first time, and smelled things and tasted things I felt I had never experienced before. It's really available to everyone but you have to open your eyes. Come to your senses. And it really put a missionary fire in me, because it was so satisfying and life-changing for me that I felt everybody should feel this way.

What was your motivation?
Alice: I wanted to taste . . . the food that I had in France. I wanted that experience. And so, I was determined. *[laughter]* I don't know where it comes from, it's just in me. And maybe it's kind of a perfectionist im-

pulse that comes from my father. It's also a desire to be liked and appreciated. It's certainly not about the fame.

You are very busy, with your restaurant, and the school lunch program in Berkeley and other projects. When it all gets to be too much, what do you do to recover?
Alice: I go to see my friends. I get acupuncture. Something that's pleasurable for me is walking and I never ever imagined that would be part of my life. If I don't do it every day, I feel disconnected from the natural world. It's kind of a centering thing. I walk a mile, run a mile every morning. Before I even wake up.

Tell us about having your daughter, Fanny (Alice married Fanny's father two years after her birth).
Alice: My parents are very close and loving and there they are, eighty-nine years old and madly in love still. But there was never a kind of openness about anything sexual . . . just because of that I felt like it was all taboo. And growing up in the fifties . . . I couldn't even tell my parents that I was pregnant. *[laughter]* I mean, Oh my god, they'll think that I had had sex. *[laughter]* But fortunately my parents thought it was wonderful. And now, my daughter is not inhibited like I was.

Did you have anybody that you really looked up to as a child? Who were your role models?
Alice: No. I mean it's very strange, I thought of professions rather than individuals.

Did you think you were going to be a chef when you were a kid?
Alice: No. I thought I was going to be a housewife. Although, *a cowboy,* that was something that I wanted to be. I always thought of myself a little bit in the men's world and I feel a bit more of a male sensibility in a funny way. There have been times when I worked in the restaurant where I just think I'm more like a man than I am a woman. I've always thought of that wonderful song in *My Fair Lady*: Why can't a woman be more like a man. And I would think why can't a man be more like a woman? The thing is, so much is about balance.

But I was really a tomboy when I was a kid.

Who are the people to whom you really look in your life for inspiration?

Alice: Lulu Peyraud—a French woman. Eighty-three years old and she's an amazing woman. Now she has a love of pleasure. *[laughter]* Richard Only wrote a book about her. He's a wonderful, wonderful cook, you should know about him, because he's a mentor of mine. Elizabeth David is another one.

There have been a lot of great women cookbook authors, but unless I'm mistaken, it seems like you're the first big female chef. Was that something that was motivating you?

Alice: No. I didn't even think about it. I just wanted to taste the food that I had in France. I wanted that experience. And so, I was determined *[laughter]*.

CHAPTER 17

Don't Be Afraid to Change Your Mind

Pleasure is forgiving

FROM CITY GIRL TO COUNTRY GIRL—MARIA

I have always said that I would live in my house on Main Street
forever. I could picture my old age perfectly—sitting on the front
porch, walking everywhere, my garden so old and gnarly that all the
dogs and cats would occasionally get lost in it. Drinking tea from my
chipped china cups. Lou and I have cared for the house and added on to
it as if resale would never be an issue and we were creating our family's
heirloom home.

Then one day Maya and I decided to go to Iceland. We'd been
reading about what a cool city Reykjavik is, but mostly I was obsessed
with going to the Blue Lagoon—a milky, powder-blue steaming hot
bath in the middle of a lava field. It was on my list of top ten things to
do before I die. Lou decided to stay home with Eve so Maya and I
went on a high school graduation trip.

I had wanted to get out and see the countryside, so we also drove to
Vik, home to black beaches and tall scary looking cliffs, about four hours
outside of the nearest city. We drove past giant waterfalls, glaciers, wild
ponies, mountains, and miles and miles of moss. It was August but the

170

weather was about 40 degrees and raining. Everything was green, though, and beautiful. I had never, ever been so far away from civilization. I felt completely myself in the middle of that emptiness.

That night as I lay my head on the pillow to go to sleep I heard a voice. It was kind of loud and booming. It reverberated inside my head and shocked the wits out of me. Believe me, I had never heard voices before! It said:

"I WANT TO MOVE."

"Huh?" I said to myself. Where did that come from? My heart was literally thudding in my chest from the surprise of it. But after a few moments, I realized it was true. Until I had stepped far, far away from the busyness of my everyday life, I couldn't hear the still, small voice inside of me. Clearly, deep in my soul I really wanted to move since that little voice had turned into a really big voice.

The next day as I lay floating in the blue lagoon, the steam and sky merging into one (it was even better than I had imagined), I realized that the voice had told me the truth. I really did want to move. I was going to move. I was going to move to the country, where the air was fresh and the loudest sound was the birds and the wind in the trees.

When I got home and told my husband about my revelation, he agreed, good man that he is. We knew we'd made the right decision when we noticed how happy Eve was when she was running in the country. When our neighbor, the hardware store, installed a propane tank right next to Eve's play set, over the fence, we *really* knew our decision was right. We saw our move as an exciting challenge, a new adventure, an opportunity to create a new life. Now, five years later, after finding some land and working with an architect, we're about to move into a new, ecologically sensitive house. There were stops and starts, second guesses and trouble all along the way, but in the process of creating our dream home I remembered something.

When I was a teenager, I had dreamed of building my own home. In those days I was actually going to do every part of it myself. I used to draw pictures of it during school. And when Lou and I first met, we talked about one day building our dream eco-home together.

I was telling this whole story to my friend Ann, as we were riding horses in the high desert of southern Colorado.

"You didn't *choose* the house you were living in on Main Street.

Now you have made a choice," she said. She was right. I had lived in that house on Main Street since getting out of high school because my mother owned it and she didn't want my sister and me living at home with her anymore. We rented it for years until my sister got married, had kids, and built her own house. Eventually I bought it so I could have more freedom to do what I wanted, but it was mostly a safe place, a place that had been there when I was young and raising a baby on my own (but close to my sister).

Once I had made my new choice to move it almost couldn't happen soon enough. I felt like I had outgrown the house, as if it were a shell or skin I was ready to shed. I had changed my mind. And I am so glad I did.

THE TRIALS AND TRIBULATIONS OF BEING A PICKY EATER—MAYA

Don't tell my mom this, but sometimes in the privacy of my own apartment I listen to Jackson Browne and Dar Williams. In fact, I'm doing it right now. And I like it. You can't tell her this because those were the songs I always *insisted* that she change if I was present. No offense to Jackson or Dar, but for a while there I just didn't get it. Naturally, my mom said if I didn't like the music I could leave the room. But sometimes, I stayed. And one time when she was at work and I was home alone I borrowed some CDs of the very music I claimed to hate.

Don't tell my mom this, either: the other night I was at a party and they served cheese and I ate it. This is scandalous because I have thrown some real temper fits when my mother even suggested that I stand within ten feet of cheese. I would refuse to eat dinner if she made something with cheese in it.

I am a notoriously picky eater. Please consult with me first if you ever invite me over to dinner I don't do cheese unless it's melted, or with wine, or if I'm in the mood. It can't be too stinky either. I don't like PB&J; in fact it makes me nauseous even to type that out. Mayonnaise is a no-no. Tomatoes are gradually being incorporated into my diet. And I don't like beans, although sometimes nowadays I will eat them with nachos. And I don't really do anything in the realm of dairy products except ice cream.

Because of my extreme pickiness as a child, my mother threw up her hands and made me pack my own lunch, even when I was six years old. Because I didn't like sandwiches, and I was only six, I often ended up with a bag of dry Cheerios for lunch, because I don't like milk.

Once, my babysitter made tuna salad sandwiches, which I hate. I wasn't allowed to leave the table until I ate it. I sat at the table all afternoon, through naptime and until my mom came to pick me up. These days one of my favorite foods is raw tuna, but I still don't like tuna salad. I am completely irrational about these things, I know.

I remember once my mother made a strange soup. [Actually, and this is her mother speaking, it was black bean soup for which I had grown the beans myself in the garden. It was pretty bad soup, though.] I refused to eat it. I was forced to sit at the table until it was time to go to my Brownie meeting. When we returned home the soup was still on the table and I was forbidden to do anything else until I ate five more bites. I cried. I gagged. These days, of course, I eat my Mom's homemade soups with pleasure.

And I say "don't tell my mom" but maybe she deserves to have an "I told you so" moment after all I put her through about food and Jackson Browne and Dar Williams. But I changed my mind and I liked it.

DO IT: CHANGE YOUR MIND ABOUT SOMETHING

Spend a quiet moment thinking. Is there something you have said or done that has left you feeling backed into a corner of your own making? In romance novels, a key plot line is the stubborn hero or heroine who has Definite Ideas about what his or her life will or won't be like. "I will not marry A Rake!" she might say. Or he will say "I will marry a nice, safe obedient woman who won't challenge me. I certainly will not marry That Hoyden." The fun is watching their stubbornness gradually crumble under the weight of their mutual desire until they are both right where they belong and exactly where they said they wouldn't be: happily in each other's arms.

LIST: MIND-CHANGING DISCOVERIES

The Earth is round! After figuring this out, countless people no longer had to worry about sailing off the edge of the world.

The Earth revolves around the Sun, not the other way around! People went to prison over this one. It was only in *1992* that the church admitted that Galileo was right about the Earth and the Sun and cleared his name of heresy, more than three hundred years later!

There was a first "Eve," or seven of them. And she was black. When a strand of DNA was extracted from the body of a man frozen for over five thousand years and tested, geneticist Bryan Sykes was called in to examine it. This led to the discovery of "a particular strand of DNA that passes unbroken through the maternal line . . . to trace our genetic makeup all the way back to prehistoric times—to seven primeval women." He calls these women, and the book detailing this theory, *The Seven Daughters of Eve.*

The Nag Hammadi Gnostic texts and Dead Sea Scrolls. Buried in jars hidden in caves for thousands of years, these biblical outtakes, released in the 1990s, shed new light on Christ, women, and spirituality.

Female reproductive and sexual organs don't wander around the body, and they don't have a negative effect on women's mental capacity. In ancient Greece any sort of illness or problem in women was attributed to hysteria, a word that means "wandering womb," which they believed got loose and floated around the body causing problems. In America, in the late 1800s, operations were performed on women to remove their ovaries or clitoris, as a cure for sexual desire and to transform them into "pure" and sexless women. Who do you want to control your body—the government, men, a society's beliefs, or you? Not coincidentally, as women have become more involved in public life, the question of reproductive rights has intensified.

The discovery of ancient Crete and Minoan culture. The discovery of the palace of Knossos and Minoan culture led to some real evidence for the existence of a peaceful, prosperous civilization where women were equal to men.

The importance of hygiene to health and medicine. It took a bunch of women—wives, mothers, and midwives—with some common sense to insist that washing hands and medical instruments with soap and water would prevent infection. It took a while for doctors to believe them.

Antibiotics. The discovery of penicillin in 1928 radically improved the treatment of many bacterial infections. Unfortunately, since it's a good thing in small doses, some people think it's a great thing in mass doses. These days most animals for slaughter (cows, pigs, chickens) are dosed with antibiotics as a "preventive" measure. Scientists and doctors have shown that too frequent use of antibiotics lessens its effectiveness on bacteria, which evolve defenses and resistance quickly. Limit your antibiotic use and eat only organic, antibiotic-free meats and dairy. And don't annoy your doctor to give you antibiotics when you have a virus. They don't work on colds and flu.

Cell phones. They sure take the worry out of kids not being home on time!

IN HER OWN VOICE: AYN RAND

"We are those who do not disconnect the values of their minds from the actions of their bodies, those who do not leave their values to empty dreams, but bring them into existence, those who give material form to thoughts, and reality to values—those who make steel, railroads and happiness. And to such among you who hate the thought of human joy, who wish to see men's life as chronic suffering and failure, who wish men to apologize for happiness—or for success, or ability, or achievement or wealth—to such among you, I am now saying: I wanted him, I had him, I was happy, I had known joy, a pure, full, guiltless joy, the joy you dread to hear confessed by any human being, the joy of which your only knowledge is in your hatred for those who are worthy of reaching it. Well, hate me then—because I have reached it."

"Isn't it wonderful that our bodies can give us so much pleasure?"

"John Galt is Prometheus who changed his mind. After centuries of being torn by vultures in payment for having brought to men the fire of the gods, he broke his chains and he withdrew his fire—until the day when men withdraw their vultures."

". . . She burst out laughing. It was a sound of triumph."

PLEASURE REVOLUTIONARY: WHO IS DAGNY TAGGART?

"Who is John Galt?" That's the first line and recurring question of Ayn Rand's massive book, *Atlas Shrugged*. The copy on the back of the tattered, often-read paperback edition that sits on my desk says it's the story about a man who sets out to stop the motor of the world. It's really about Dagny Taggart.

A fictional heroine who runs a transcontinental railroad, Dagny is a beautiful woman, not only because of her looks, but because of her intelligence, ideas, confidence, hard work, and values. Bad guys are scared of her, but good men *love* her. She runs the family railroad business at a time when America is falling to pieces, when the men in charge pass laws to thwart her goals of profit and productivity, when truly visionary businessmen disappear one by one, making Dagny's job that much harder. While everything collapses around her, she stands with her head held high and says, "I give the orders. I am right, I know that because of the logic, and reason, because I trust and value my own brain."

When I was in the ninth grade, my mom handed me a tattered paperback copy of *Atlas Shrugged*. For one week I did nothing but read it, I could do nothing else. I had found a heroine who was smart, competent, and had great love affairs with great men. She was my ideal. People mocked me, "Oh, Ayn Rand, you don't believe that stuff, do you?" "It's a good story," I said, with a shrug. A lot of people don't read Rand because her work has been adopted by conservative Republicans, many of whom read it because it supports their policies. But you can read it in two ways. The first is to see it as any orgy of capitalism. A refugee from communist Russia, Ayn Rand believed that envy and jealousy were at the root of communism—the sense that if one person had something good, all should share. To some communists, it was even better for no one to have anything good, because excellence draws too much attention to an individual.

But you can also read *Atlas Shrugged* as a quintessential woman's story. I first liked it because I was concentrating on the love story. Dagny is virtually the only strong female heroine in a canonical novel who does not suffer in the end for her passions. She works her way to the top. She succeeds despite those around her who hate her for it. When I started writing this piece one afternoon, I picked up that old copy, just to glance at the novel. At three in the morning I forced myself to put the book down and get some sleep. I woke up five hours later and kept reading. Within twenty-four hours I had reread it—again.

"There is no *give*," says John Galt. It's true, Ayn Rand doesn't believe in altruism or handouts, on getting something just because you need it. Instead, she earns everything she gets. Remember, as the characters do, your first paycheck. I think that Ayn Rand is trying to say that we feel great personal satisfaction in earning something, and that pleasure in productivity is the motor of the world.

Dagny and her great friends are actually fighting for happiness—the kind that comes from knowing you've earned it. While the bad guys in the novel exalt suffering, they are terrified by intelligent, competent, happily independent people refusing to suffer, people who are "incapable of the conception that joy is a sin." The losing guys say "Pleasure is not an essential of existence." The heroes reject that limited view and look for joy in personal accomplishments, their own minds and intellect, sex, business, and quiet moments alone.

For the first eight hundred pages, John Galt is just a figure of speech, uttered in times of despair. He is linked to the motor of the world—he's not only stopping it, he invented it, and he is somehow involved in the mysterious disappearance of the thinking men. He is the mysterious "destroyer" Dagny has sworn to kill, the invisible obstacle in her way. Naturally, they fall in love.

"Why does he fight his hardest battle against the woman he loves?" asks the front page of the book. The heroes' refrain is, "Check your premises. There are no contradictions." Dagny eventually understands, about 950 pages into the book, checks all her premises, and changes her mind. She does not give up what she values, but comes to understand that she can change her tactics without selling out—without giving up what she knows is right, or herself. She can "swear by my life and my love of it that I will never live for the sake of another man, nor ask another man to live for mine."

And that's when she gets her happily-ever-after—the love of a hero who understands and respect her, as well as her own sense of satisfaction with herself and her accomplishments. After 1,084 pages, she has earned the reward for her passion.

~⁓~

CHAPTER 18

Delegate and Negotiate

Pleasure is not a tyrant or a martyr

MAN IN THE HOUSE—MARIA

Men have always resisted having women in "their" workplace. But gradually, we are gaining access and working our way up, proving that we can do it. If we can't do things their way, then we do them our way—which is different. I have a theory that women are just as territorial about their place—the home—resisting quietly and angrily any infringement of men into their sacred domain.

I discovered this theory one night while I was doing the dishes, seething in my own martyrdom. In my head the conversation was going something like this: My husband and I both have jobs. We both work full time and in fact overtime. It's not fair that he gets to come home and watch sports on TV while I make dinner, do the dishes, take care of all the kid stuff, *and* change the light bulbs, call the repairmen, and write the checks to all the people who come and go from our house.

We were newly married at the time, so I was just following the example of my own martyr of a mother. More often than not when Lou did try to help out around the house, I would just get mad because he didn't do it "my way" or as well as I would have done it. He'd do the dishes but he wouldn't wipe the counter. He'd complain about how the house didn't feel like it was his—but when he suggested changes I would find a reason not to like them. Plus, he was extremely sensitive to anything that sounded like "bossing" on my part, and on principle passively resisted my dictatorship.

So I'm doing the dishes and I'm thinking about all this and suddenly I realize that I've got to let him in. Sure, I could do it all—but why would I want to? If I was going to have equality at work, I had to have it at home, too.

So I called a family meeting, kids included. Together, we made a list of all the chores in the whole house, inside and out. We went around the table, each of us picking the ones we preferred to do. By the time we got to the bottom of the list we all had equally odious things we had to do that we didn't enjoy. It felt fair.

The clincher was that now I had to let Lou do it. I had to let him do the dishes his way, in his own good time. Were they done every night before we went to bed? No. Is the trash taken out every week? No. Is the lawn mowed and trimmed nicely every week? No. Every two weeks? Sometimes. But like a little kid learning for the first time, I tried to encourage rather than complain. I am still learning how to ask for things without sounding like I'm being bossy. But I have also learned not to let it get to me (as much). Those things are his job, not mine. And if I really need something done for some reason I ask nicely.

Delegating the chores has freed me, too. If I don't feel like making dinner, I don't. If the house is especially messy I can now ignore it. Do I love everything perfectly clean? YES! But I also know it only lasts for a brief moment in time and then it gets messy again. I'd rather spend my time doing something fun with my family, or creating something, or reading a good book.

The unexpected consequence of my letting Lou in is that now he's a real partner and a real good dad, too. I can easily leave on a trip for business or pleasure knowing that Eve will be safe and well taken care of while I'm gone. She may not have home-cooked meals or get to bed on time, but she will have fun. He's had a major influence on the whole design of our dream house. It's his as much as it's mine.

Not long ago I tried to read a *New York Times* best seller called

Bitch in the House. I loved the one essay written by my friend, Cynthia Kling, but the book kept bringing me back to that time, that feeling when I felt I was the only one who could do it right and I was mad as hell that Lou wouldn't do it my way. *Everything* got better when I got over that. Now, instead of a bitch in the house I've got a MAN in the house. I highly recommend it.

LITTLE MISS DICTATOR—MAYA

At one point senior year of high school, I was in complete control. I was the editor-in-chief of the school newspaper; founding editor and writer of the underground school newspaper; class vice president, which meant organizing the senior skit (a horrific task); I was in charge of the radio club; I was organizing the annual battle of the bands, as well as rehearsing with my own band for the monthly open mic nights that I had co-founded. Oh, yeah, I had classes and was applying to college. On a few occasions, I had to leave class to go cry in the bathroom.

Some of the work I created for myself and really loved, like the newspapers and the battle of the bands. Other jobs were handed to me saying, "If anyone can do this, you can, Maya." I had earned myself a reputation, and I was determined to live up to it.

Organizing projects, and especially people, is an art. It's like sculpting without being able to see the clay until the finished product is on stage with a spotlight in front of hundreds of people (if you're lucky). It is at once terrifying and exciting. Besides the long hours and not being able to visualize the end result, the really hard work is having to deal with people. Male musicians, at least the ones I knew, are difficult because they just want to jam for hours on end without a thought to the audience or the logistics of getting them onstage with equipment. Each guitarist had his own special amp. Every singer needed to be a little louder. Lighting the stage, soundchecks, and getting apathetic high school students to come watch were all tough. As the resident dictator, I oversaw every detail, from securing the April date in September to making posters to hang up all over school.

When you're a leader, acting like a plan is brilliant when you have your doubts is the most stressful and important aspect, even more than attending to details or making decisions. Which is why I went to cry alone in the bathroom. No one could see me do that.

I had a reputation to live up to, a persona I had created for myself. Suddenly, in the quiet of the girl's bathroom, I admitted that maybe I had taken on more than I could handle. A list of my extracurricular activities could barely fit on the one page required for college applications. After the applications were in the mail, I took a look at my schedule and decided what really mattered to me. I gave some other kids the chance to fill up their afternoons, rather than act as dictator on almost all school projects.

Certain things I kept for myself as long as I could, including the annual battle of the bands which I had started and starred in for three years. One of my last acts as a senior in high school was writing out step-by-step, month-by-month directions on how to bring the whole event together. I made a few copies, stuffed them into envelopes and gave them to the two younger students I felt were most capable. I found out a year or two later that the event was still going strong. Sometimes, I like to read the copy of instructions I kept for myself, remembering all the effort I would put into that one night. Organizing a huge event is tremendously rewarding, but not as much as sleeping for two whole days when it's over.

DO IT: MAKE A LIST, DIVIDE AND CONQUER

If you live with others: Call a meeting when everyone is in a fairly good frame of mind: well fed, well rested, and not in a rush to go somewhere. Sit at a table with a tablet, pens, stickers, whatever you like to use for scheduling. Explain the new situation and how it's going to be a new day in the house, where everyone is equally involved and invested in running the household. Be open to criticism and complaints, but don't let them get you sidetracked. Together, make a list of all the household chores. Go around the room and let everyone pick the ones he or she prefers to do. Then divide the less appealing ones equally among you. Let people trade and negotiate with each other—you are the referee and ultimate authority, however, so don't hesitate to "lay down the law." Try not to nag people about doing their stuff. But also realize they may not know how to do it right and may need your guidance.

If you would like more help, read *Just Kiss Me and Tell Me You Did the Laundry*, by Karen Bouris. The book has a step-by-step process you can follow.

If you live alone: you should still make the list of all the things you have to do. Are there some you can hire out? Can you afford a cleaning person or accountant? Try to find alternatives to the things you loathe. For example, if you hate making the bed, just don't do it! Or get a pretty comforter to throw over the rumpled sheets and pillows to hide them. (I have to confess, our beds get made once a week, when the cleaning lady changes the sheets.)

Note to everyone: In the pantheon of household chores there are those that HAVE to get done and those that would be nice if they are done. Make sure you focus first on the essential ones, and relax your standards on the optional ones.

LIST: TOP TEN REASONS WOMEN DON'T GET WHAT THEY WANT

We suffer in silence. Historically, women who have spoken up have been scorned—as much by other women as by men. We probably carry that tendency to deny a problem inside of ourselves. Who hasn't said, "I'm fine" when something wasn't fine? Enough is enough. Every opinion, idea, or feeling that you don't express holds you back. No one is a mind reader, but most people are capable of listening. So say something.

We fight among ourselves. It took over a hundred years for women to get the right to vote in this country. Perhaps part of that was due to bickering, disagreements, and gossip among the early suffragettes. Put a common goal ahead of petty competitions. What legacy do you want to leave for your daughters? A personal feud, or a positive change in the world?

We think we don't deserve it. Historically, women have been told we don't deserve success, freedom, equal rights. Women have been told throughout time that we're not even capable of learning. And millions of women have proved this wrong. If you work for something, you earn it, and you deserve it.

We don't ask for a raise. The average woman still earns around eighty cents to every dollar that a man earns in the same profession. Maybe it's because we don't ask for the raise we know we deserve.

We blame "The Man" for holding us back. It isn't all the men's fault. Successful women, like our Pleasure Revolutionaries, accomplished so much in much harsher environments for women. With determination and hard work, they didn't let anyone or anything hold them back—not men, or laws, or disdain from other women.

We get bogged down in housework. There are always dirty dishes, floors, and laundry, despite our best (OK, sometimes half-hearted) efforts. Menial chores often take up time we could spend doing something we really love. If you have kids, a significant other, or a roommate, delegate the chores. Try not to let your place be a mess when you go to bed. For me, Maya, doing dishes when I'm dead-tired, or putting my clothes away before bed is worth it because I wake up in a clean apartment in the morning, with my time free to do what I enjoy. [This is where Maya and I part ways. At the end of the day I don't care about the mess and I just want to plop into an unmade bed with a good book.]

We try to do it all because it is "expected" and not because we want to. Women are now expected to advance our careers, be supermoms, wives, and girlfriends, exercise regularly, eat right, and keep a clean house. Yet there is a definite trend of working mothers giving up trying to have it all, quitting their jobs to be full-time moms. These women decided what they wanted and what their priorities were, and then went for it. Decide what really matters to you, and then find a way to make it happen.

IN HER OWN VOICE: QUEEN ELIZABETH

"There is only one Christ Jesus and one faith: the rest is a dispute about trifles."

"A realm gains more in one year's peace than by ten years of war . . . no war, my lords!"

"I will have here but one mistress and no master."

"Though I be a woman, yet I have as good a courage, answerable to my place, as ever my father had. . . . I will never be by violence constrained to do anything. I thank God I am endued with such qualities, that if I were turned out of the realm in my petticoat, I were able to live in any place in Christendom."

"Little man, little man, the word *must* is not to be used to princes [me]."

PLEASURE REVOLUTIONARY: QUEEN ELIZABETH

Never let it be said that a woman can't lead a country. The rein of Elizabeth I was an unprecedented, perhaps unequaled, forty-five years of peace, prosperity, and devoted leadership, from 1558 to 1603, the Golden Age of England. Don't even pretend that it was easy.

The almost cartoon-like image of Elizabeth many of us hold in our heads—red wig, white painted face, and unnaturally high forehead—is mostly a figment of the Hollywood imagination, which portrayed her virginity as a marketing ploy to appease her people. The real queen is so much more complicated and remarkable.

Elizabeth's mother, Anne Boleyn, had her head chopped off when Elizabeth was three, in 1536. Years later, one of her favorite step-mothers, Henry's fifth wife, also was guillotined. You would think this would have made Elizabeth hate her father, King Henry VIII, but in fact she adored him. Even though she was third in line after her elder stepsister Mary and brother Edward, she was raised from the first to be a queen, and was baptized a Protestant, and crowned when she was twenty-five in 1558.

Extremely intelligent, Elizabeth spoke many languages, was good with numbers and even frugal, and had a fine grasp of human nature. No frail bluestocking, she loved to ride horses extremely fast, dance like crazy, and adorn herself with jewels and silk stockings. She also loved to take baths. To the public, she was serene, steadfast, and always in control—but in the privacy of her own court, she often let her nerves get to her. She loved her job, her country, and her people more than anything.

She surrounded herself with smart, loyal advisers who stuck with her until their deaths. Her favorite, by far, was Robert Dudley, the earl of Leicester, who was handsome, loved to dance, was an expert jouster, and was passionate about horses. Elizabeth made him Master of the Horse, and some historians believe she also made him her lover. Nothing can be proved, but clearly they were both passionate about each other and exchanged many romantic, intimate letters and gifts.

Her council and subjects all expected her to marry and have heirs. Marriage was also seen by her advisers as a way to control her abundant energy. One smart Scotsman summed it up, "Your Majesty thinks that if you were married you would be but Queen of England, and now you are both King and Queen. I know your spirit cannot endure a commander." She craftily used her "betrothability" to her country's advantage to keep her England out of war, cultivating long-term potential alliances with France. While she loved to flirt and was very susceptible to the affections of handsome men, she never did marry—she feared the suppression of her power in a marriage, feared childbirth (which was almost a death sentence back then), and loved Robert Dudley.

While pretending an interest in marriage, Elizabeth reformed England's currency, built the most powerful and fastest shipping fleet in the world (they called her "Queen of the Sea"), got her country out of debt, encouraged the adventures of Sir Francis Drake, the first Englishman to sail around the world, and supported the arts, including Shakespeare's first plays. Yet through thirty years of her reign, she fought off the continued assault of the Scots for their claim to the throne led by her cousin, Mary, Queen of Scots.

Mary, Queen of Scots, had the support of the Catholic Church, which ruled Spain at the time. In 1570, the pope actually issued a proclamation stating that Catholics living in England "shall not once dare to obey her [Elizabeth, who had been baptized a Protestant] or any of her laws, directions or commands." (This is the same pope who made a medal commemorating the slaughter of hundreds of Protestants and Huguenots in France on St. Bartholomew's Eve.) A cardinal in Spain actually sanctioned Elizabeth's assassination by saying that since she "is the cause of such injury to the Catholic faith and loss of so many million souls, there is no doubt that whosoever sends her out of the world with the pious intention of doing God service, not only does not sin, but gains merit."

But Elizabeth's popularity was so great, and Mary, Queen of Scots, so distrusted, that even the majority of the Catholics in England would much rather enjoy peace than war and supported Elizabeth. The only time England went to war was when Spain dared attack England. Elizabeth took herself to the front lines in armor and made an impassioned speech to her troops, declaring: "I know I have the body of a weak, feeble woman but I have the heart and stomach of a king, and a king of England too, and think foul scorn that Parma or Spain or any prince in Europe should dare to invade the borders of my realm." The Spanish armada was so soundly defeated by the English Navy that they never even touched land. When the news of Spain's defeat was announced in a Jesuit school in Rome, many of the English students were heard to shout with joy. The people loved Elizabeth, because Elizabeth loved them.

After thirty years of scheming, Mary, Queen of Scots, was finally accused of treason and beheaded in 1587, a decision that pained Elizabeth greatly. She never once sent someone to the executioner's block without great regret and often spent days mourning their deaths.

One by one, Elizabeth's devoted council passed away from old age, which saddened her deeply. The world was getting more complicated, and she was getting tired. At one of her final council meetings, she said, "It is my desire to live nor reign no longer than my life and reign shall be for your good." She was sixty-nine, and died of natural causes soon after.

Elizabeth was born on the eve of the Feast of the Nativity of the Virgin. She died on the Eve of the Feast of the Annunciation of the Blessed Virgin. Her motto was: *Semper eadem*—Be always one.

CHAPTER 19

Set Goals, Visualize Success, and Reward Yourself

There is pleasure in accomplishment; celebrate success

THE LILY OF THE FIELD—MARIA

*B*ack when I was a hardworking nine-to-five girl I took the advice of some business magazine to "dress for the next job you want." Off I went, pleased to have an excuse finally to justify my taste for fine clothing. A few people close to me seemed to disapprove of my extravagance (not Maya!). I did it anyway, all the while picturing in my head the kind of life I wanted to have.

Years later, I've honed this skill to an art. I am currently dressed for the job I want, which is the job I have: a writer. The ideal outfit consists of being unshowered and naked underneath a serviceable bathrobe with some flip-flops. I still love fine clothes and now I can afford them. My reward is that I don't have to wear them if I don't feel like it.

I was in the car one day with Lou explaining my theory to him—a sort of "if you build it they will come" theory: Spend your energy visualizing what you want, set goals to get there, and then reward yourself when you achieve any of them (and reward the universe by being generous with what you have earned). Lou worries about money a lot, and at the time he was worried about the money we were spending to build our new house. Humble living is a virtue to which he aspires. While I love that about him (and it reassures me he didn't marry me for my money), it also is a point of contention sometimes since I basically believe that when I work hard and reach goals it's OK to reward myself by spending money. In fact, the less I worry about money, the more it seems to come to me. Because I'm working hard and enjoying myself, it's fine if I get money, it's fine if I don't. I don't feel guilty for wearing fine clothes and building a big house. I worked for it and had faith that my work would be rewarded. Plus, the more money I make, the more I am able to give it away to others who need it more than we do.

I suddenly connected this to Jesus' teaching about the lilies of the field. "And can any of you by worrying add a single hour to your span of life? And why do you worry about clothing? Consider the lilies of the field, how they grow; they neither toil nor spin, yet I tell you, even Solomon in all his glory was not clothed like one of these" (Matthew 6:27–29). The universe and nature provides for the lilies' survival and beauty. So many religions (and their followers) seem to demonize money, passion, lust, beauty, success, and desire. But those things are not inherently bad. What we do with them and how we use them makes them harmful or good. Picture the lily of the field, gorgeous, fragrant, perfectly beautiful. It's her faith in nature that sustains her, so even when she shrivels and dies at the end of the season she knows she will rise again.

And so I continue to conjure up a world I want to live in. I visualize the goals I need to achieve to create that world and take time out to appreciate the rewards. The rewards are sometimes financial—my new house, my not having to worry about this month's bills (although I put in my time doing that over the years!). Sometimes the rewards are physical—a massage, a good meal, an afternoon nap. Sometimes the rewards are adventures—trips to places I've dreamed of going and exploring. And I don't feel guilty about any of it. Do you think a lily ever felt guilty? No. Maybe she even felt glorious. She probably felt sexy, too.

But I also know the best rewards don't cost a thing: Snuggling on the couch with my little girl and breathing in the fragrance of her skin (otherwise known as sniffing her neck). Enjoying a peaceful, loving partnership with my husband (and getting him to laugh!). Having a house that's a pleasure to come home to because it's a haven of love. And at the end of the day a really comfortable bed.

THE LITTLE THINGS AND MY MIU MIU BOOTS—MAYA

After all my activities in high school, I was burned out. So the only extracurricular activities I attempted during my first two years of college involved beer, boys, and instant messaging. My first semester in New York, I had more free time than I knew what to do with. I didn't have many friends just yet, and didn't bother to join any clubs. So that summer, I decided it was time to take advantage of all the city had to offer and get an internship and a job.

I found a listing online for an internship at *Interview* magazine. I filled out the application, and sent it off along with a sparse resume and some writing samples. A friend of the family put in a good word for me at a trendy downtown restaurant, since with essentially no work experience, I was having a hard time finding a job. Once a week, this restaurant had open interviews. So I went once a week for three weeks. Even with my connection, I still had to stalk them. September was fast approaching and I was getting hopeless.

My mom came into the city for a day, as she often does. Since I was unemployed, I had all the time in the world to follow her around, and I followed her all the way to the Miu Miu store in SoHo. There, I fell in love, hard and fast, with boots that I just knew had my name on them. They were like black leather motorcycle boots, with two metal clasps on each, and the trendy pointy toe. Most importantly, they had very low heels. Because if there is one thing I had learned in New York by that point, it's that only the ladies that can afford to take cabs *everywhere* wear the stiletto shoes made popular by *Sex and the City*. As I was unemployed, cabs everywhere were not an option. Plus, I liked walking around the city. And these boots were comfortable and stylish and I *had* to have them. They were also five hundred dollars.

So my darling mum and I struck a deal. If I got the internship, that was one shoe. If I got the job at the restaurant, that was another shoe. I despaired and I dreamed and I saved my money, because it was looking like if I wanted them, I would have to buy them both.

And then one day my phone rang. It was Rich from *Interview*, calling to schedule an interview. And just as I was plotting the perfect outfit, and calling my mom at work to tell her I had earned a shoe, Rich from the restaurant called, basically hiring me over the phone. I called my mom back telling her those boots were mine.

I got the internship and the job. I just needed the boots. I went back to the SoHo store and they didn't have them in my size. I went to the uptown store on Madison Avenue and they didn't have my size either. I ended up having them shipped in from a store in L.A. Size 5s are hard to come by.

They arrived at the end of August when it was still too hot to wear anything but flip-flops. I kept them in the box until it was cool enough to wear them. And wear them I did indeed, each step a reminder of what I had done to earn them, until the heel was worn away, and the metal base made clicking sounds on the sidewalk with every step I took. I brought them into a shoe repair place and the man behind the counter gave me a look like, "Gee, lady, what did you do to these shoes?" But he fixed them. And when I was busy seven days a week going to college and working at a magazine, and working in a restaurant, those boots were with me every step of the way.

DO IT: BE YOUR OWN CEO—SET A SMALL GOAL AND GIVE YOURSELF A SMALL REWARD

It doesn't have to be momentous (like losing twenty pounds or finding a new husband). It can be small, but significant. Maybe you got through one day without screaming at your kids. Or you exercised once this week. You made one really good, healthy home-cooked meal. Or you came to a tough but important decision.

We are both firm believers in the value of New Year's resolutions and daily lists. Crossing things off those lists can feel like its own reward, but we like to reward ourselves even more tangibly than that. We call it incentive-ising yourself. It's human nature. It's also good business management. So now you can live your life like you are your own CEO. Work hard and enjoy the rewards.

One of the biggest and best rewards that you can give yourself— and one that most CEOs overlook—is rest. Take naps occasionally, take time off, make time just to sit and reflect—these are actually essential to your health and your success. Often in those quiet moments, the best ideas and thoughts come. That's why people tend to get ideas in the shower. When your mind is turned off and forced to be quiet, you can actually hear the universe talking.

LIST: THE BEST REWARDS FOR YOURSELF

Take a nap. I (Maya) am forbidden to call home on the weekends between noon and four, because most likely, the family is napping. It's not an issue anymore, because I too now take naps then. There is something so wonderfully simple about crawling into bed in the afternoon and saying "I'll wake up when I wake up."

Read a romance novel or watch a romantic comedy. They are fun, smart, and sexy. And best of all, you don't feel any stress wondering how it's going to end. Studies have shown that movies like these are far more relaxing than other genres for the very reason critics scoff at them—the formula and guaranteed happy ending allow the brain to go on "auto pilot."

Read "trashy" gossip magazines. We call them "brain candy." They are light, relaxing, and occupy the mind without overstimulating when you need a break. And don't feel guilty about it: Recent studies show that the impulse to gossip was once a survival tactic; it was a way to distinguish friends from enemies. *Psychology Today* refers to a study that found that "teens who keep up to date on celebrity gossip are popular, with strong social networks—the interest in pop culture indicates a healthy drive for independence from parents."

Buy yourself flowers. One friend of mine says having fresh flowers on the table is not an indulgence, but a necessity. They're beautiful, they smell good, and every time you look at them, it's a reminder that you care about yourself and your home.

If you always cook, get take out, or vice versa. Do something differently than usual. No matter how simple, it can be exciting and feel like a treat. Taking time to enjoy a good meal gives you a feeling of satisfaction beyond just feeling full.

Buy something you really want. Save up, go visit it in the store, and then treat yourself and buy it. Bring it home to love it. I have a pair of earrings that I bought as a treat for myself when I got my first raise. I love them because they're pretty, but also because I feel I've earned the right to own and wear them. Besides, buying stuff helps the economy.

Have a spa treatment. It's not necessary to spend a lot of money on it.. You can buy products to use at home. Often just taking time to care for your own body feels great. But if you do go to a spa, enjoy having someone else attend to you.

Challenge yourself with something totally different. When was the last time you went for a bike ride? Or visited a small, but interesting local museum? Find something near by you have never done or seen before and give it a go.

Be a sloth for a day. For two days after my college graduation, I did nothing but read romance novels in bed. Sometimes I play computer solitaire for hours on end (after I get my work done, of course). Some-times, I watch TV all day. Sometimes I don't even bother to get dressed. Something about being a complete sloth rekindles my desire to be productive.

Go to the movies by yourself. Lots of people do it, so don't be scared. The plus sides are that (1) you don't have to share the popcorn, (2) there is no one to bother you by talking to you during the movie, and (3) you don't have to compromise on what movie you go to see or where you sit.

Pat yourself on the back. Acknowledge to yourself that you did some-thing you're proud of. Savor the feeling.

Listen to music. It's hard to imagine that up until about a hundred years ago, if you wanted to hear music you had to hear it live. Now you can listen to any kind of music from all around the world. Music can soothe you, comfort you, pump you up, and get you moving. We highly recommend satellite radio for crystal-clear, static-free, and mostly advertising-free listening exploration. Plus, it tells you who the artist is so you can buy the CD or download the song.

The world is a wonderful place.

IN THEIR OWN VOICES: VENUS AND SERENA WILLIAMS

SERENA

Favorite place to visit: the mirror in her house

Biggest goal in life is to win Wimbledon [she did it!]

VENUS

Favorite place: anywhere that accepts credit cards

Life goal: to avoid further speeding violations

⁓

"I plan EVERYTHING around my outfits."

VENUS

"We're not perfect but we work hard and have fun and we're attractive and strong and have high standards."

VENUS

"I hate losing, so that drives me to win. When I [lose], it's not the best feeling in the world, but I get over it."

SERENA

PLEASURE REVOLUTIONARIES: VENUS AND SERENA WILLIAMS—THE WINNING SISTERS

It wasn't that long ago that women just didn't play sports unless they were outcasts—their reputations were already ruined so it didn't matter. At best, a proper lady could become a good horsewoman. In the last hundred years or so a few women have gradually risen in the pantheon of sports: Peggy Fleming in the 1968 Olympics; Billie Jean King, the tennis star who beat Bobby Riggs in the first prime-time male-female match in the 1970s. Greta Waitz, nine-time winner of the New York City Marathon, tells a funny story about her first New York marathon. Even though she won, she says she was really there because her husband wanted to run. She not only didn't know what a marathon was, she didn't realize how long it was and spent most of the time running cursing her husband for making her do it.

Sometime in the 1980s, little girls started playing soccer. Little girls started to believe they could do whatever they wanted. Little girls realized they didn't have to stop running, playing, and enjoying the strength of their bodies to "settle down." They could keep playing and win. In this fertile ground of sports possibilities, Venus and Serena were born. They were raised to play tennis and have won basically any-thing and everything there is to win in the world of women's tennis.

Right after their dad saw Virginia Ruzici win the French Open in the 1970s and get a check for around $22,000 (100,000 francs), he vowed that all of his unborn children would play tennis. In 1984, "Richard loads four-year-old Venus, six rackets and seven milk crates full of tennis balls into his Volkswagen van and travels to the public courts in Watts and Compton, where he gives his daughters lessons. 'It's a radical neighborhood,' Richard says of the area around East Compton park. 'A lot of dope is sold.'" By 1990 the *New York Times* does a story featuring Venus with the headline: "Status: Undefeated. Future: Rosy. Age: 10."

Since then, both Venus and Serena have won the French Open doubles—and became the first sisters ever to win a Grand Slam crown together. They have each won Wimbledon and the U.S. Open. They each have won Olympic Gold Medals in the 2000 Sydney games. In 2000 Venus was named sportswoman of the year by *Sports Illustrated*. In 2002 Venus became the first African-American woman to reach the number one ranking on the WTA Tour. Now, with endorsements from companies like Nike and McDonalds, the sisters are wealthy beyond their wildest dreams. In fact, Serena has been declared the richest woman athlete in the world.

Since they are both only in their early twenties it would be easy to imagine them turning wild and self-destructive. But they seem to have a firm grounding in their faith and both are pursuing more creative careers. Venus is studying to be an interior decorator and Serena is planning on becoming a fashion designer. In fact, her courage on the court extends to wearing shockingly nontraditional outfits while she competes. That's just one of the many reasons we think they are true Pleasure Revolutionaries.

CHAPTER 20

Expect Satisfaction.
Ask for It

Pleasure believes that sex is good

SWIMMING IN THE SEA OF LOVE—MARIA

To me, sex is like the ocean and we are in a boat. From the deck of the boat, the ocean seems terrifying—especially if you have no idea what's under it. The surface is dark and turbulent. Strange sea monsters leap out of it. Its tides and storms toss us about. As much as we try to close our eyes and ignore it, the ocean is there and in fact we need it. We need it to define the shore. We need it to keep us afloat. We need it to eat. The planet needs it in order to survive.

Now imagine we are on a big boat with lots of people and all the kids are asking "What's that thing out there called? Can I touch it?" And the parents say "Oh, that's nothing. Don't even look at it. And especially don't touch it! That's bad!" So the kids grow up knowing the ocean is there, feeling it with every sway of the boat. They kind of like it because it's comforting, but they feel guilty because they've been told it's bad and they shouldn't know about it. Occasionally one of the parents sneak off for a swim, shameful and embarrassed at their momentary need. But they have perfected the art of pretending it never happened.

Now imagine for the first time you can scuba dive and you go under. Suddenly there is a whole new world right beneath you, surrounding you. The scary things that looked like sea monsters are giant, loving, peaceful whales. Yes, there are bad things down there . . . sharks and shipwrecks and strange tides that pull us in the wrong direction. But knowing is power. Understanding makes you appreciate the whole beauty and complexity of life. Suddenly, you love the ocean and feel it has been a part of you since the beginning of time. And you realize that the scariest part—like waiting in a doctor's office for a test result—is *not knowing*.

The world has for some inexplicable reason made sexual "not knowing"—ignorance—into an art. I know lots of people who will let their kids play violent video games and watch bloody movies but won't let them anywhere near naked bodies or sexual knowledge. (Just think of the Janet Jackson Super Bowl uproar: It's fine for small kids and grown ups to watch hours of grown men crushing each other and piling on top of one another, and companies pay a fortune to advertise during it, but the sight of one nipple has the whole country in a hysterical frenzy). This is not new. In *The History of Sex* documentary by the History Channel, there is a story about John Ruskin, a famous author of the 1800s whose only knowledge of sexuality and nakedness was from seeing ancient marble roman statues. When he married and found out his wife, Effie Gray had hair "down there" he was utterly disgusted and refused to sleep with her. It took her six years to figure out a celibate marriage was not normal, and she finally had the marriage annulled. She went on to have a passionate love match with a new husband, the artist Robert Millet.

A fascinating book called *Technology of Orgasm*, by Rachel Maines, documents the invention of the vibrator in the late 1800s. In the Victorian era, doctors and nurses used the vibrator to help them with the time-consuming manual duty of bringing women to orgasm to cure the symptoms of hysteria, a female syndrome, which included "volatile emotions, overdramatic behavior, and susceptibility to suggestion," according to the *Oxford English Dictionary*, and was epidemic. Sexual ignorance was so widespread that even doctors did not know that women, as well as men, had sexual needs. Eventually, doctors invented all sorts of tools for relieving women's pent-up sexual frustration in order to get them to "paroxysms," or what we call today, orgasm.

Medical masturbation goes all the way back to Hippocrates and Celsus in the first century A.D. In 1653 a medical text provided a similar remedy for hysteria that midwives could practice on "widows, those who live chaste lives, and female religious."

It took me a long time to get over my own guilt about my sexuality. I did a lot of reading, exploring, and experimenting before I came to terms with my own desires. One of the things that helped me the most was watching TV, especially the PBS series *The Secret Life of Plants* and the PBS series on *Evolution*. I was fascinated to find out (being a gardener) that basically flowers and nature are all about sex. Some flowers mimic exactly bee vaginas. We are constantly surrounded by a buzzing, hissing, growing, ever-expanding mass of fornication, because without sex, there is no life. The desire for sex is the desire for creation, procreation, continuation, and faith in our future. The intermingling of sperm and egg to create new life ensures the genetic diversity of our species . . . and our survival. Plus, it's fun. It reduces stress and eliminates the disease of hysteria (I do believe I know some women who still suffer from it today). We are the only species (that we know of) that gets so much pleasure out of sex—long after our eggs have dried up. We are also the only species that has a pleasure center (clitoris) separate from the procreation center (vagina). We were made for pleasure, and without it we get sick.

The sad thing is the unknowing and ignorance about female sexuality and our own potential for sexual pleasure continues. In 2004 the *New York Times Magazine* had an article on the new trend in the "Bible Belt" of sex toy parties. Many women who show up have never had an orgasm. Some don't even know they have a clitoris and what it's for. The woman who runs these parties has a euphemism for the clitoris to keep embarrassment levels manageable: She calls it "the little man in the boat."

Ladies . . . it's time to dive in.

THE BEST THIRTEEN DOLLARS I EVER SPENT—MAYA

In my senior year of high school, a friend and I skipped a free period and drove to the Gothic Erotica store in a near-by strip mall. Newly eighteen, we showed our driver's licenses to the clerk and were admitted to the back room, the one with all the porno and vibrators. We each picked out a waterproof pocket rocket for $12.99. The best thirteen dollars I ever spent.

Shortly thereafter, in the safety of my room, I had my first orgasm. Then a few more. I was a teenager, I had hormones, and for lord's sake, if my options were high school boys or a battery operated device, there was really only one choice to make. I bought my satisfaction, and it was worth every penny.

Packing for college, I debated whether or not to bring it. I figured I wouldn't be needing it anymore, and I didn't want to leave it at home to be discovered. So I threw it away. And let's just say, there were many nights that first year of college that I thought, "Damn, that was a dumb thing to do, throwing away my vibrator."

Two years went by before I got another. By then, I was living in New York. With the boys I was seeing, I knew it was time to get another one. One of my friends decided that she too wanted one, so off we went to the West Village, where there are about ninety-five stores selling all sorts of sexual toys on every block. We went into the first one. Under a glass case, I saw another "pocket rocket." It was pale pink. "That's kind of like what I had before," I told her. "Did it work?" she asked. Yeah. Yeah it did.

But just in case, we asked to try it—on the palm of our hands. The sales girl unlocked the glass case and screeched to some guy on the other side of the store, "Chang, we need a demo!" My friend and I were kind of mortified as this guy brought over a single AA battery. We got our demo, and made our purchase. These cost thirty dollars; apparently orgasms in New York are more expensive. We both agreed later that we had made the right decision. She even named hers.

One day, years later, mine broke. I thought maybe the battery had died, and so I ransacked every remote control and every other AA battery-operated device in my apartment. But it was clear that it had died. So I threw away one more vibrator, and couldn't imagine a life without another.

I went alone, this time to Toys in Babeland, a store for girls. Instead of the usual sex-shop atmosphere of bad lighting, stuffed with giant dildos and creepy old men, this one was . . . nice. The store was well-lit and had a rosy glow. The merchandise was well-organized and presented neatly and cleanly. Just walking into this store was exciting. And there they had my trustworthy pocket rocket, only this time in many different colors. For a moment, I was overcome and I thought I wouldn't be able to make a choice. I bought one in hot pink.

DO IT: ASK FOR SOMETHING YOU REALLY WANT, OR GIVE IT TO YOURSELF

This year, if anyone asks you what you want for the holidays or a birthday, give them something specific to buy for you. It doesn't have to be sexual, but it can be. And then, if you don't get what you want, buy it for yourself.

Sometimes asking isn't enough to get you what you want—your desires might be different or in conflict with your partner's or whomever you are asking. Don't sulk if that's the case, at least you asked and now you know! Then, go out and get it for yourself.

LIST: BEST SOURCES FOR GIRL TOYS, PORN, EROTICA . . . THAT SORT OF THING

You can get all sorts of sex toys almost anywhere these days. But if you're not interested in smutty shops with bad lighting, and prefer discreet shopping and shipping, check out these websites. The thing that separates them from other sex peddlers is their emphasis on a woman's pleasure, without shame.

Toys in Babeland / babeland.com. Oh, my, this place is amazing. They advocate safe sex with love and fun and toys for girls! On the website, they sell all sorts of products, books, DVDs and offer tips and advice for better, more pleasurable sex. They have in-store workshops. Basically, anything you could want or need for better sex (except for a partner) is available at Toys in Babeland, shame free.

Mypleasure.com. While this website is geared toward women, their extensive selection offers toys for men and toys for couples as well. They also offer guides and tips. Check out their "Sex Toy Timeline," because, hey, it's educational.

Sh! Women's erotic emporium. This London-based store won't even let men in unless accompanied by a woman, lest their presence compromise their "relaxed, nonjudgmental atmosphere." If you're not in the city, you can check out their website, Sh-womanstore.com, where they too provide sex tips with sex toys.

Emotionalbliss.com. It calls itself "the site for sexual happiness" and offers quizzes, the opportunity to talk with a "sexologist," and erotic stories and products.

Edenfantasy.com. More sex toys, and not just for women. This site in particular has lots of links to related sites, like **womensporno.com**, a porn site devoted to images pleasing to women.

Goodvibes.com. This San Francisco–based woman-owned company is one of the pioneers in sexual pleasure. It's a great source for toys, advice, videos, and just about anything you could wish for when it comes to finding immediate satisfaction.

Sex.com. Go ahead and explore the giant universe of porn. There are lots of sights that give you free peeks and you get a real insight into human nature. Whatever your pleasure is, however kinky or strange, you will be reassured that there are lots of others just like you.

Just one warning: When you start visiting porn sites, you are susceptible to getting internet viruses that can junk up your computer with pop-up windows and spam. So use protection—have up-to-date anti-virus software.

IN HER OWN VOICE: THE THUNDER, PERFECT MIND*— SHOCKING WORDS FROM LONG AGO

For I am the first and the last.
I am the honored one and the scorned one.
I am the whore and the holy one.
I am the wife and the virgin.
I am the mother and the daughter.

---

* "The Thunder, Perfect Mind," dated approximately 300 B.C.E to A.D. 400, is a Gnostic text that does not fit into any known religious tradition.

 The quote shown is an excerpt from a longer poem that was published in *The Other Bible* (Harper/Harper Row), originally from the Nag Hammadi Library, 1977. The translator is George W. Macrae. Some believe it is similar to other texts relating to Isis, the Egyptian name of the Great Goddess. The speaker is powerful in her transcendence, and its origins are mysterious.

I am the members of my mother.
I am the barren one
And many are her sons.
I am she whose wedding is great,
And I have not taken a husband.
I am the midwife and she who does not bear.
I am the solace of my labor pains.
I am the bride and the bridegroom
And it is my husband who begot me.
I am the silence that is incomprehensible
And the idea whose remembrance is frequent.
I am the voice whose sound is manifold
And the word whose appearance is multiple
I am the utterance of my name.

PLEASURE REVOLUTIONARY: INANNA— THE ORIGINAL SEX GODDESS

Who is Inanna? Her story starts in an ancient time, when the world worshipped the Great Goddess, the Queen of Heaven, from India and Iraq to the British Isles (before they were British). Then, the mother goddess was revered around the world. She was the original It-Girl. Inanna was just one of her names, her Sumerian name. She is Ishtar in Babylonia, Isis in Egypt, in the Bible she is referred to as Astarte and Ashtoreth. She is Aphrodite in Greece, and Kali-Ma in India. They are all different names of the goddess of goddesses, world shakti, or female spirit of the universe. She is the Mother of the World. She lives on today as the Virgin Mary, the mother, and Mary Magdalene, the lover. According to The Thunder, Perfect Mind, she is "the whore and the holy one, the first and the last." A contradiction? Perhaps it's time to check our premises.

By whatever name you choose to call her, Inanna was a three-faced goddess, which some scholars believe to be the basis of the Christian trinity. She was seen as a virgin, mother, and crone; the creator, pre-server, and destroyer. Her sacrament was sacred sex, and for that she had priestesses at her temple, often called temple prostitutes, who received money for the temple in exchange for sex. The priestess was perceived, and treated, as the earthly incarnation of the Goddess. Sex between the priestess and a male worshipper wasn't any old wham-bam-thank-you-ma'am fornicating. They believed they were imitating the ultimate act of creation, by uniting the male and female aspects of the universe and themselves, as well as with The Divine. It was the ultimate ménage à trois. There was no threat of rejection, no shame in the pleasures of two bodies. Sex was a humanizing, civilizing force. They made love in honor of something holy. It may have been like the steamy sex scenes in romance novels, where the female and male physically and metaphorically become one, and their differences are not sources of conflict, but pleasure. A line from the wedding hymn for the sacred marriage was "Oh my queen, queen of the universe, the queen who encompasses the universe, may he [the king] enjoy long days at your holy lap."

The Goddess was also about fertility of the people and the land. She was the bride, and the king was her bridegroom. She had a son or brother/lover—sometimes they were the same—who was ritually sacrificed each year. Her consort was Damuzi (or Tammuz) and her virgin-born son was named Attis. Each year, her consort was ritually sacrificed—his blood needed to fertilize the land. And each year, as women wept and wailed for the death of the man, the Goddess descended into the underworld to revive her love, and this resurrection ensured the fertility of the land. This is the story of Isis and Osiris, of Cybele and Attis, and even of Jesus. This is the story of the cycles of the moon, of the changing seasons, of winter turning to spring. Innana was the source of the earth's life force. Water was her blood, and any source of water was sacred to her.

The Goddess is Mama. This one syllable, MA, is the sound that many a baby first utters. It is found in the name Kali-Ma, from India, the Greek goddess Demeter (meter is Greek for mother). MA is also an Egyptian pictograph for the spark of Life, and in the Iranian moon-goddess Mah. MA is said to mean "a state of immortality brought about by drinking the milk of the Goddess's breast."

Women can tap into the powerful attributes of the Goddess: her sexuality, creativity, sensuality, and her natural force. Her force is also our force. We have the power to be creators and preservers and destroyers. We, too, can be like the true, original meaning of the word virgin—She Who Is One Unto Herself. Satisfaction Guaranteed.

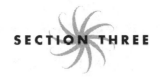

Live the Life You Have Always Desired

YOU HAVE FOUND YOURSELF, IF ONLY FOR A MOMENT. You've done the hard work to conjure, visualize, and create the life you have always dreamed of. Now it's time to live it. Live it in the big ways. Live it in the small ways. You can live a life of pleasure even when times are bad—and you can truly appreciate the times that are good. Live your pleasure every day.

It's time for you to become the author of your own story. No one else can write it for you. Sure, maybe someone else set the scene or determined a few early characters. But you and only you can decide whether yours will be a tragedy or a romantic comedy, a long boring literary challenge or a thrilling page-turner. You are responsible for the story of your life.

You alone have the power to decide your legacy. Will you leave the world—your world—a better place? Or leave a wake of chaos and pain behind? Will you heal the relationships in your life, and your own pain? Or create even more hurt and let your own hurt fester?

You are unleashed. You are an adventuress. You are strong. You are a healer. You are a pleasure revolutionary.

THE THIRD FACE OF THE GODDESS

The Crone

The third face of the Goddess is perhaps the most misunderstood. She's a wise woman but is often seen as a witch. She is each of us after we go through menopause, when our estrogen decreases, our testosterone increases, and our assertiveness and energy soar. Our hormones free us from our maternal role. We are no longer as bound to our children—or even our husbands if we choose. We are free to become our true selves and explore the meaning of our lives. We have the courage of the warrior and the power of the destroyer. We can choose to stay asleep in our routines until we die, or to waken anew and spend the twilight of our life giving back to the world and ourselves.

The crone is autumn and winter. She embodies the beautiful decay of a blazing colorful tree whose leaves are falling, falling, falling until the essential bones of the tree are fully exposed, ready to start a new season in her life.

CHAPTER 21

Travel Alone

Pleasure and life begin and end alone

GRAMA AND NANA WENT TO JAPAN TOGETHER AND DIDN'T SPEAK TO EACH OTHER FOR TWENTY YEARS. I GO ANYWHERE . . . ALONE—MARIA

Both of my grandmothers were widowed most of the time I knew them. During my growing up they were both wonderful sanctuaries, each a very different sort whom I loved to visit. But even I knew at a young age that they didn't get along well. They would be fairly polite to each other when they were both invited over, but you never knew what might happen. Fortunately, because one grandmother was Jewish, she didn't have to attend all the Christian holidays we celebrated in our house, and so we avoided some potential fireworks.

My mother's mother—Grama Harter—as I called her, was a lady through and through. Her house was a veritable gift shop of paperweights, little animal figurines, old books of poetry, and china teacups. Towards the end of her life she would pound her cane and say with pride, "We were *French Huguenots*!" But mostly she was "Pennsylvania Dutch." She never learned to drive, so for approximately forty years she stayed mainly in her house.

My father's mother—Nana—was a creative fury. Unleashed when she was widowed in her sixties, she'd tear around in her Cadillac, mink coat, and Hush Puppies. She opened a restaurant, a bookstore and gift shop, and traveled to Africa, Europe, and Iran on buying sprees. She had an apartment in New York City, which she would drive to in her big car, always stopping right before the entrance to the New Jersey Turnpike to pull a china cup and saucer, a linen napkin, and a thermos of black coffee out of a wicker basket in the trunk to fortify herself for the final part of the drive. She was truly a coal miner's daughter, had a fifth-grade education, and was orphaned at age twelve. She moved to Manhattan when she was fourteen, married well a few years later, and converted to Judaism reluctantly to please my grandfather. She was a modernist painter, and her house was like a dusty treasure chest that was constantly rifled through. Usually, something was bubbling on the stove that smelled good, although sometimes chicken's feet were sticking out of the top. When I was finally old enough to notice my grandmothers' long-running, seething feud, I asked my mother what had happened, since by all accounts it was Nana's and Grama's friendship that originally brought my parents together.

"Well," she began. "Nana and Grama decided to go to Japan together on a tour. Apparently they were on a bus and the bus was going on some very windy and scary road. Nana was nervous (and probably carsick) and asked Grama to please be quiet. When Grama wouldn't shut up, Nana smacked her." Apparently they didn't speak to each other for the rest of the trip, or forever after except for the bare necessities. Grama never traveled again. Nana kept going . . . either alone or later with her grandkids, who would shut up when she told them to.

I decided that I was going to be more like Nana in her spirit of adventure, but more like Grama in her manners. And I was going to travel alone.

My first big trip alone is a point of controversy between Maya and me since I missed her first birthday. She is rightfully appalled. I feel I have a reasonable excuse.

Between the ages of nineteen and twenty-one, my life radically changed. At eighteen, I was a high school graduate with no plans, no place to live, no stuff (other than an inky old typewriter and some Indian bedspreads), a boyfriend I was ready to break up with, and no real direction. By my twenty-first birthday I was the mother of an almost-one-year-old with an apartment filled with baby and housewarming gifts, and a thirty-seven-year-old boyfriend. I was enrolled in a local college and somehow I had accumulated all this stuff. I had never been to a bar (legally). I didn't know who I really was anymore. I had overwhelming cravings to go to the desert.

So over spring break (Maya's first birthday) I went to New Mexico. We had a big party for her before I left and she got plenty of presents. After I left, she stayed with my parents, whom she adored. But I had to go find myself. I went to Santa Fe and Taos. I stayed in a room Georgia O'Keeffe had lived in for a while. I painted. I went to a bar and got really drunk and almost slept with an even older man. I spent the next day grotesquely hung over. I missed Maya desperately. And when I gladly came home I can't say I had found myself yet, but I knew now what was truly important— Maya, and me. I spent the next few years painting the desert.

Since then I have traveled alone a lot, sometimes for pleasure, lots of times for business, enjoying every single cup of room service coffee drunk in bed. Once I even slept on top of a mesa without a tent, and watched shooting starts fall all around me—the ultimate fulfillment of my desert fantasies.

Now that I know that I can travel on my own, the whole world has opened up for me. And I'm not waiting to be a widow to enjoy it.

BECOME WHO YOU ARE—MAYA

I ran off to Paris when I was nineteen looking for love, life, and adventure. As if I was the first person to ever think of this. But all of us expatriates and escapists know that we are really looking for ourselves.

When I was a kid my mother would drag me to what I called "women finding themselves movies." They were always period films, and women would leave their dull lives and duller husbands and take lovers while on holiday in Italy or other picturesque locations. Somewhere along the way, they would figure things out: they would remember who they are, who that person is "deep down in the secret velvet of your heart, far beyond your name and address," as one of my favorite authors described it. I don't remember the specifics or names of any of these movies, but the theme became permanently lodged inside. I loathed them . . . until I lived my own version.

Off Rue Mouffetard, in the area where Hemingway lived during *A Moveable Feast*, I had a single room, on a classic ancient cobblestone street. Old ladies walked it with their shopping carts. It had an open-air market, restaurants, and bars—lots of bars. I sat in cafés at the Place Contrascarpe, writing where Hemingway had sat and probably looked out at the same fountain, which seemed as if it had been there for a thousand years. When I wasn't lolling about in cafés, I was taking classes in French art and film. Except for other students I met, I had traveled to Paris alone.

When I arrived in Paris, I was jaded. I was bored. Life was a chore. But there was something about Paris—the light, the air, that *je ne sais quoi*, something so seductive I couldn't resist it. Within days I was in love—merely being alive became magical and mysterious again, like the body of a new lover. Every sidewalk was the greatest, the most perfect that I had ever walked on. Every cup of black coffee, every little French puppy, every cobblestone street, every ride on the Metro—I was in love with all of it. I could hardly contain my laughter while I walked down the street, thinking to myself, "This is so ridiculous. This is my life."

So far, it was just like the movies: Girl leaves monotonous homeland for the exciting life abroad. But that was only the first step. I was just like Christian from *Moulin Rouge*, coming to Paris to experience beauty, truth, freedom, and above all, love. The second step is: fall in love with life, then you can fall in love with a boy. Become completely lost in another to find your true self.

I called him Prometheus because he always had a light for my smoke. He was a student as well, an American. I had intended to have my affair with an indigenous Frenchman, but this boy was It instead. I was too happy to argue. Our first kiss happened sometime late, late at night, or very, very early in the morning. We sat side by side on my bed, with the window open to the soft morning light seeping in and the last drops of a rainy night lingering in the atmosphere. We sipped cheap red wine straight from the bottle. He was the one to kiss me. I had one condition: "What happens in Paris stays in Paris." Prometheus had a high-school sweetheart back home; I was the Other Woman.

I became his mistress, his *belle fille*. The French word for mistress is *maitress*, which sounds like *maitre*—master. When I was younger, I was obsessed with the idea of being a mistress. It seemed like the most romantic way for a woman to retain her autonomy yet still have a committed, passionate affair. From the stories I'd read, the men with mistresses were kings and aristocrats. Prometheus was neither of these, but I didn't care. This was my big opportunity. I walked around like Madame Bovary thinking, "I have a lover! I have a lover!" with exclamation points and all.

I settled into my new life, the one I had always dreamed of, the one I had lived in my head before I fell asleep at night. Fantasy had become real. My days were a pleasurable ritual, one that I would have lived out every day for the rest of my life, if I could have. I would wake up next to Prometheus, in his room with a view of the Pantheon. I had breakfast at a particular sidewalk café at Place Contrascarpe, where the waiter had learned what I wanted. He brought my espresso with a glass of cold water, and with a small piece of chocolate. No one else got such treatment, and I never even had to ask for it. I rode the Metro to school, over the Seine and past the Eiffel Tower. In between classes, I would linger in the courtyard and pull out a cigarette to attract Prometheus and his lighter. I spent the afternoon in the cool of museums, staring up at Manet's *Olympia* or the *Venus de Milo*.

Evenings were spent in the local bar, the Fifth, full of other students. There were three bartenders—Kaise from Scandinavia, Mark from South Africa, and Lauren from the States. Ragi from Norway was always there, as was a wandering guitar player, and Earl, a dirty old man who owned our other favorite drinking place, called Shebeen. We drank liters of beer for fifty francs and smoked *gauloises*, which came in packs of thirty cigs. We shared stories of trying to speak to the locals, or of people we knew back home. It was the expat atmosphere I had longed for. I became one of the regulars, one of the locals for six glorious weeks.

One night, getting bored of the usual bar hopping, Prometheus and I took his guitar, exactly like the one I had left at home, out to the open square at Place Monge. It was chilly, after midnight, and the streets were empty, except for drunk couples on their way home. He and I took turns playing songs for each other—songs I had written for past boys, songs he had written for the girlfriend. He said he wanted to be a boy in my songs, but I wanted him to be different from all the others. Hearing him sing about his girlfriend made me want to cry and throw up. But as the Mistress, I sang along, for the final song, the one we both knew, the one with the chorus of "my aim is true."

The next afternoon I took myself out for a late lunch at the Hotel Costes, off the Rue Saint Honoré. And here everything came together. I was confidently alone at nineteen, in a foreign country, far from the safety of home, in a hip restaurant, ordering in French, smoking my cigarette, writing it all down. I had made it on my own and learned how to be alone. I was living a fantasy life—and had become who I wanted to be.

The third step of the finding-myself movie—the trip was over. The torrid love affair was finished, but while it had "broken her heart, it has opened her mind," as one author wrote. I told Prometheus I never wanted to see him again; I was done being a Mistress. It was time to go home, time to come back from the edge. This was where the movie ended but the rest of the story had only begun. I didn't mind going home because it wouldn't be the same home I had left; I would be living my life with a new point of view.

Sitting on the floor of the Paris airport, I wrote that I was far from home, with nothing to show for myself except for a suitcase full of dirty clothes, a broken heart, and dark roots showing through my blonde hair. But that is everything. It's the evidence of adventure.

DO IT: YOUR FIRST SOLO TRIP—
HOW TO DO IT AND LOVE IT

Decide where it is you, and you alone, want to go. Maybe there is a faraway place that everyone has teased you for wanting to go to. Now imagine yourself traveling there alone. This is your trip. Pick it. No one else has to agree with you or approve.

If you are afraid, you may want to make your first trip alone a day trip, or join a tour group. There are many tour groups or study-abroad programs to join up with. As long as you don't go with anyone you already know, you will have the freedom to be who you've always wanted to be, as well as meet lots of new people who will probably speak your language.

As you travel alone, you'll find that you'll get inside your head like never before. You're going to see and feel and experience things with a wonderful intensity. You'll also be able to do whatever you want without having to compromise with travel companions. This is a wonderful thing.

Not scared yet? Good, then you're ready to start. Actually, it's normal to be scared. Don't let that stop you.

If you can't afford to go some place far away, go some place close. The point is to be out there on your own, satisfying your own wanderlust and no one else's. Test your own limits of risk and adventure. You can do it. And, yes, it's a pleasure. And yes, yes, yes, you are strong and free.

LIST: WHAT TO PACK

When traveling as a woman alone, it's a good idea to pack for both safety and adventure. This list will get you started.

Knowledge. It's always helpful to know where you're going and a little bit about the place. Read guide books and magazine articles, even novels that are set at your destination. It's also helpful to learn a little bit of the language: hello, goodbye, please, thank you, and where are the bathrooms? And check the weather! The first time we went to Paris in the summer, we packed warm weather clothes, and it turned out to be freezing. So now every picture from that trip is of us wearing the only warm outfit that we each brought.

Safety stuff. Let's face it, some places are safer than others for traveling alone. But still, you are going to have to protect yourself. If you are in a city, learn which neighborhoods are safe. Read up on local customs and behavior so you can blend in more easily (and be less of a target) and so you don't accidentally do something offensive. One of the most important safety tips is to dress conservatively and according to the local culture. If you are in Paris in shorts, sneakers, and a T-shirt you are a target. Don't tell people that you're traveling alone. Always keep a map in your bag, but if you have to look at it, try to go into a ladies room rather than stand on the street corner. Hold onto your handbag. And trust your instincts—if something doesn't feel right, remove yourself from the situation. And wherever you go, don't drink the water unless you know it's safe: buy it bottled. It can be scary and a downer to think of these things, but it will ultimately make for a better trip.

Wishes. What do you want to do while you're away? Are there particular landmarks you want to see, or restaurants you want to try? Perhaps you don't want to make any firm plans but simply wander around. This is good, too. Is there something in particular that you're looking for? Make your wish list and don't leave home without it.

Clothes. The two most essential things: a good pair of walking shoes and underwear. It just wouldn't be fun to spend your whole vacation walking around with blisters while shopping for underwear. Anything else you forget, you can just buy when you get there.

Recording devices. Cameras, pens, paper, sketchbook, your own memory. Bring something that will allow you to capture your memories and thoughts and feelings. We find that keeping our travel journal is a great thing to do while dining alone, which you're going to have to do if you travel alone.

Empty space. By that we mean an extra suitcase. Because really, is there any place left in the world that doesn't have something for sale and something to buy?

An adventuress attitude. Last, but certainly not least, when traveling alone it's all up to you whether you have a fun, exciting, life-changing trip, or a solitary pity party in a foreign country. It's up to you to get out of your hotel room, and off into the world. Did you ever wonder why the crabby, complaining people seem always to have the worst things happen to them? Being nice is a universal language. Having patience and persistence will get you through almost anything.

IN HER OWN VOICE: JANE DIGBY, FEARLESS TRAVELER

"Forgive me, dearest Lewis, if our last night's conversation pained you, but your openness, affection and sincerity encourage mine.

It is not to be denied that rapture, *untasted for six months*, has [now] reawakened passions I have flattered myself were nearly if not quite extinguished. Still, dearest, I repeat my *intentions* remain unchanged. . . . My word of honour I regard as a sacred vow and I dare not, dare not, give it lightly."

"The sword dance, where men and women joined, I thought graceful, and pleased me as more characteristic of their manners . . . we joined in . . . to the *delight* of the Bedouins and though I felt a sort of shyness steal over me in the presence of so many, I knew that if I chose I could surpass them all in fire and agility."

"Saturday April 3rd. My birthday. Sixty-two years of age and an impetuous, romantic girl of seventeen cannot exceed me in ardent and passionate feelings."

PLEASURE REVOLUTIONARY: JANE DIGBY— ADVENTURESS AND LOVER

A biography of Jane Digby is entitled *A Scandalous Life*. This beautiful, smart Englishwoman was a great adventuress, and followed her heart all over the world from the lush English countryside to a hot Middle Eastern desert, living a life filled with princes, kings, and sheiks.

Born in 1807 to an admiral father and a mother declared to be "the handsomest woman in England" by the Prince Regent himself, she lived with her family on her grandfather's estate. Thomas Coke was one of the richest, most powerful "commoners" in England, and even turned down the offer to join the peerage. The Digbys had hoped for a boy but adored the beautiful, charming baby Jane who arrived instead. As a child, Jane preferred racing horses with her brothers to playing with dolls. She shared their lessons as well, and developed a fondness for history and a fluency in multiple languages.

Nicknamed "the light of day," Jane came of age in the Regency period, in which many a romance novel takes place. After just one season of dinner parties and soirees at Almacks (the famed "marriage mart"), she made her match and at seventeen married a prominent lawyer, Lord Ellenborough, who was about twice her age. Soon after the wedding, however, the husband who had exchanged love poems with his wife turned out to be a philanderer. Jane was often left alone in London, socializing with a crowd much older than herself. Perhaps that led to her affair with her cousin George Anson, on whom she had

had a lifelong crush. Their affair didn't last, and the child, presumed to have been his, to whom Jane gave birth, also died a few years later.

In 1828 she met Prince Felix Schwarzenberg, the visiting ambassador from Austria. Young, heartbroken, ignored by her husband, Jane quickly fell in love, and practically flaunted the affair that would result in the birth of a daughter, one of the biggest scandals of the day, and Jane's subsequent exile. Upon discovering her adultery, Lord Ellenborough filed for divorce, which was highly unusual at a time when perhaps one or two a year were granted—and all the more remarkable since Ellenborough had previously condemned the king's right to a divorce. The divorce proceedings were a public trial, covered in all the papers, and everyone attended but Jane, who had already taken off for Europe and offered no defense. Lord Ellenborough got his divorce: Jane lost her reputation but gained her freedom.

Prince Felix, who had encouraged his young mistress to abandon everything, then abandoned Jane. While she was in Paris with him and their child, he falsely accused her of betraying him and took off. Yet through the years he would write her letters that led her on regarding his affections.

To make a new life for herself, Jane went to Germany, where she was constantly courted by Baron Carl "Charles" Venningen, a good friend for whom Jane did not feel the grand passion she wanted. She became friendly with King Ludwig I and his court, and, pregnant again, the father unclear, she married the baron, had two children with him, and for a time lived isolated in his country house.

At a party one evening, however, she met a Greek count, Spiros Theotoky, and began a passionate love affair. After much drama, including duels between the count and the baron, and midnight attempts to flee the country (and her husband and children), Jane got her second divorce and was free to travel anywhere, except Germany. She took off for Greece with her new lover and soon-to-be husband, although the baron remained faithful to her until his death.

Jane gave birth to her sixth child, a boy. While she had not felt any maternal love or tenderness for her previous five children, she fell in love with her little Leonidas right away, becoming a happily married mother at last. All went well for a few years until she caught her husband cheating. After yet another divorce, and a disastrous trip to Italy where six-year-old Leonidas fell to his death before her eyes, Jane went back to Athens alone, built a grand house, had a love affair or two, but otherwise lived alone.

Jane decided to visit "sites of antiquity" and in 1853 went to the Middle East. In her full European dress of corsets and full skirts, she engaged a guide and, with her maid, set off to tour Jerusalem and other biblical sites, in particular, the desert oasis of Palmyra. Her escort, Medjuel el Mezrab, was a Bedouin sheik in his late twenties; Jane was by that time in her forties. They set off on horseback through the desert with Medjuel's Bedouin tribe. For the next few years Jane would travel through the desert, return briefly to England and Greece, and always go back to the Middle East, for she and Medjuel had fallen in love.

In 1854, Jane moved to Damascus and built a house. She learned Arabic, adopted many Arab customs, and impressed Medjuel's tribe with her horsemanship and gift at handling their rare breed of Arabian horses. She and Medjuel fell more and more in love and wanted to marry, but Medjuel was already married and Jane would not consent to being one of many wives. Medjuel divorced his first wife, although his culture disapproved, and swore to be monogamous to Jane. In 1855 they married and set off for a honeymoon in Palmyra.

As Jane Digby el Mezrab, beloved wife of a Bedouin sheik, she traveled the desert, riding high-spirited Arabian horses by her husband's side, earning the love and respect of both the men and women of the tribe. She entertained foreign visitors, kept up correspondence with her family in England, and enjoyed the grand passion she had always longed for.

She died in 1881, at the age of seventy-four. At the foot of her grave in Damascus lies a large block of pink desert limestone, carried from Palmyra, "where Jane spent the happiest days of her life." Medjuel himself carved her name into the rock. He never remarried.

CHAPTER 22

Face the Dark Times

Pleasure has the power to heal

THE BLACK MOMENT—MARIA

Every good romance has what is fondly called "the black moment." It's that part of the book where all seems lost. The heroine is about to be raped by the evil villain and the hero has just been locked in an inescapable prison. It seems humanly impossible that they will ever be able to get back together again and have their happy ending. The black moment is often accompanied by what Dr. Pamela Regis, in her book *A Natural History of the Romance*, calls "ritual death." The hero or heroine or sometimes both are knocked out, or they're at death's door, or in a feverish delirium. Only the power of their love for each other can revive them. It's the romantic resurrection.

Real life is filled with black moments. Just because Maya and I believe in love and pleasure doesn't mean we are in denial about pain. She and I—and I'm sure you, too—have had our share of black moments. Here are some of mine: on the day I finished my last exam in college, two days before Christmas, I went to check on my brother in the hospital and found out he was dead of AIDS (only three days after his diagnosis). The next day, Christmas Eve, the man who I thought was my true love rejected me *again*. The following week, I was scheduled to move to Washington, D.C. Death, grief, loss, graduation, rejection, and moving all in one week.

Or another day, I had to tell my mother as she woke from anesthesia that she had breast cancer. Then I had to call my dad at his regular lunch to tell him, too. And one beautiful, sunny fall day my sister had to call me into her office to tell me that our father had been killed in a car accident. In Moscow. I woke up for weeks afterwards, every morning, remembering all over again and crying.

Despite all our differences, my dad was still one of my best friends. I think one of the reasons that my father picked me as his business heir is my strength under pressure. When tragedy happens, I go into robo-mode, which does make some people uncomfortable, since they expect to see more emotion. I spent the day I learned of my father's death making sure everyone else was informed and accounted for. I told my mother. I tracked down my brother, who was fairly determined not to be found (it took a few hours). I picked up Maya from school and told her (that was the hardest part of all). I made dinner for all the people who showed up at my mother's house. I made sure the coffee pot was filled and picked the wine from the wine cellar. Then, in the quiet of my own room, in my own house, I broke down and cried.

Seven years later, as I was on my way to the supermarket to pick up food for nine in-laws who were arriving for the weekend, I pulled into an emergency medical center because I thought I was having a heart attack. The business unit I was running was going to lose four million dollars with no hope of recovery; my art director who had recently arrived from New York City had just been diagnosed with Hodgkin's disease and was wasting away on chemotherapy; and my mother and I were preparing to fire people who had been at the company longer than I had been alive. Turned out I "only" had heartburn.

Although in time I recovered from those deaths and resolved the business issues, I sank into a depression so deep and dark that my emotional brain kept saying I should just kill myself even though my logical brain knew I had every reason to live and knew things would get better. I loved my kids and husband desperately but couldn't seem to pull out of the dive.

My depression ended when I went to Japan, in March of 2001. Seriously, the minute I entered the Tokyo airport I was cured. That's not as strange as it sounds, because I have since learned from Dr. Helen Fisher that doing novel things raises dopamine levels, which lowers depression. Going to Japan with two kids and with none of us knowing a word of Japanese, either spoken or read, was certainly novel. And it was better than drugs as far as I'm concerned. I don't want to anesthetize or numb myself from my pain and suffering. I want to get to the root of it and resolve it. My depression, I believe, was the result of having gone through many personal and work traumas without taking the time to rest, recover, take care of myself, and follow my *own* dreams. Plus, I had taken personally the venom aimed at me from ex-employees and the media. A wonderful therapist helped me put it all into perspective.

Then came September 11, a black moment for the whole country. I watched it live on TV that morning, on the phone with my husband, who had been on his way into Manhattan and called to find out why all the traffic was turning around. When the buildings collapsed, I wanted to know . . . I had to know . . . where does all that hatred come from and how can it be stopped?

So I read, I researched, I questioned. How did our culture of violence start? I read books by Riane Eisler and Alice Miller, who has studied the childhoods and lives of people like Hitler, Saddam Hussein, and even George W. Bush. As Riane says, the root of violence is emotional as well as physical scarcity and trauma. Many violent people were either physically, emotionally, or sexually abused as children, although that itself is not enough to turn someone into an "evildoer." Along with that has to go a lack of emotional nourishment. No love. No warmth. No comfort. From unending black moments comes a rage so deep that a person can't contain it. Terrorism is the natural result of children who have grown up terrorized, sometimes by their own families, sometimes at the hands of other people or countries. Just as in the romance novels, the only thing that can stop the violence is love. Peace starts at home, by raising children who are loved and cared for and not abused in any way—by their parents, their community, or their country.

I know I will have more black moments in my life. Any death is a black moment. And death is inevitable. But seeing death up close and facing it has made me realize all the more how precious life is—and how important the little pleasures are that we experience from day to day: the sweet scent of autumn air, the warmth of a child or lover (or a kitten) close by, the sight of a beautiful landscape or the sound of music. Most importantly, it's taught me the power of love.

Whatever awaits us after we die—paradise or eternal darkness—I am determined to enjoy and take care of what we have right here, right now. Because, truly, life is amazing.

STREET SMARTS FOR WOMEN—MAYA

These days, women can pretty much achieve whatever they want with hard work and determination. We can get a good education, pursue careers we want, find the relationships we want, and live the life we want to live. Except for one thing: we can't walk around freely and fearlessly.

I feel the streets are the final frontier, maybe because I'm small (a quarter-inch shy of five feet) and maybe because I'm a girl. I have to spend money on a cab ride home late at night instead of walking, when a man can save his money and walk home. I don't think this fear comes from living in a city—in New York, I know which streets are well-lit and busy at all hours of the night, and feel safer than I did on my college campus in Connecticut, when walking home from the library necessitated walking through empty dark fields, with big trees and bleachers and buildings casting ominous shadows over everything. Perhaps I am just paranoid, but every morning when I read the paper, headlines declare my worst fears have happened to someone else.

Even in the daylight, a girl walking down the street can face an ordeal. I can't count how many times some guy gave me a "How you doin'," or "Miss, miss, let me just talk to you." I have had strange men follow me. I have even been hissed at. I am so tempted to turn around and say, "Oh, you're the man I've been waiting for my whole life. Nothing turns me on like being hissed at!" I want to stop and demand an apology, I want to tell them doing that is offensive and intrusive. But the last thing I want is to provoke someone. Who knows who has a gun these days? Instead, I follow the rules of dog training: the ultimate punishment for bad behavior is to be ignored.

I used to think it was my fault that I constantly attracted comments.

I started dressing more conservatively; no short skirts or low-cut shirts. And still! I have walked down the street hung over, dressed in a dirty, unflattering sweatshirt and baggy jeans, and still gotten hassled. Then I wish I could projectile vomit at will on men who comment, follow, and harass. We all, men and women, check out other people on the street. That is not the issue. I know not to take it personally, but that doesn't mean it doesn't make my heart beat faster with fear, it doesn't mean that I am not afraid, it doesn't mean that it doesn't bother me. It's not my fault, but I still feel the pain.

In period romance novels, no real lady would even think of going out without an escort or two. It must have been a little stifling, but I can understand the culture. Only when I walk down the street with a man am I immune to comments and gestures. This means harassment is not even about the girl, but the girl who appears to be alone. Of course, I don't let a lack of an escort keep me from walking around. I consider late night cab fare well-spent money. In fact, my ritual before I go out at night is to make sure I've got ten bucks stuck in my "this is not beer money" pocket.

An article about Jack Kerouac, the *On The Road* hero for millions of teenagers dreaming of escape, quoted a letter by a woman who wrote that men could have adventures, grand literary classic adventures, but girls had misadventures. A strange man following us in the subway is a misadventure.

We women have to be careful of more than just strangers. Studies have shown that 10 to 50 percent of women are victims of intimate violence. It breaks my heart to think of all the women too afraid and ashamed to tell anyone. Who is a girl to trust? Herself, ourselves. We've got to trust our instincts, have cab fare and self-defense classes, watch our drinks at a bar, watch out for our girlfriends, speak up and take action when we see something isn't right. And we've got to surround ourselves with those we can love and trust, who will watch out for us as we look out for them.

DO IT: ELIMINATE THE HATE AND VIOLENCE IN YOUR LIFE

This is a big one with major, major positive consequences, that you can't even fathom until you have tried. It's not always easy to do, but making the commitment will ease your way.

First, *forgo the scary, violent movies and TV shows.* By watching them you perpetuate violence in your own life, and you are supporting an industry that exploits violence and rage. We are not advocating regulations or rules to eliminate these shows. We are, after all, Ayn Randian, free-market capitalists. Use your own dollars and your time to make the market respond.

Second, stop violence in your own home. *Don't spank, tease, hit, or speak meanly to anyone in your home.* And don't allow people to speak meanly to you or tease or physically hurt you. If you are being emotionally, physically, or sexually abused, get out and get help—for your sake and your children's. If you are being abusive to others, get out and get help.

Third, if you are feeling an excess amount of anger or hatred, *seek professional help to sort it out,* for the sake of your own health and family harmony. Most often, that hate and rage started with a deep hurt. Without addressing the deep hurt, you will never heal. You cannot be angry and healthy. Anger and hatred physically harm your body, your heart, and mind. Without healing you will never be truly happy with your self and your life.

Healing is possible.

LIST: ORGANIZATIONS THAT ARE THERE TO HELP YOU NOW (FROM VDAY.ORG)

- If you need immediate police or medical attention, call: 911
- National Domestic Violence Hotline: 800-799-7233
- Rape, Abuse & Incest National Network (RAINN): 800-656-HOPE

IN HER OWN VOICE: NORA ROBERTS—THE BEST-SELLING AUTHOR OF ALL TIME

"Shoes are one of the things that separate us from the animals. It proves that we are a higher being. Otherwise, we could be a golden retriever. They don't wear shoes or accessorize."

"You can't have too many earrings. They are like orgasms. You can never have too many."

"A day without fries is like a day without an orgasm."

"I want to die at age 120 at my keyboard after having great sex. Wouldn't that be great?"

PLEASURE REVOLUTIONARY: NORA ROBERTS RUNS OUT OF CHOCOLATE IN A SNOWSTORM

As Nora Roberts tells it, we owe her writing career to a blizzard in 1979 that trapped her in her house with two sons under the age of six and a "dwindling supply of chocolate." In an attempt to amuse herself, and to keep from going crazy, she started writing down stories that she had been making up in her head. A few rejection letters and a year later, the newly founded Silhouette publishing company launched her career. "My sons were three and six when I started writing," she writes in *The Official Nora Roberts Companion*, a book put together by her fans. "They grew up with it—they had no choice. Writing allowed me to stay at home with my kids and make a living, a luxury few people manage. I thank my sons, Dan and Jason, for learning the vital rule of a writing household: Don't bother me unless it's blood or fire. And, as they grew more responsible, arterial blood and active fire."

Her fans call themselves "Noraholics." Many of them stalk bookstores for any new release. Fortunately they don't usually have to wait too long, since Nora is prolific and writes an average of eight books a year. She also writes mysteries under the pseudonym J. D. Robb. Her books are funny, tough, nail-biting page-turners. Sometimes they are quite violent, but the hero and heroine always save the day. "My heroine may have problems, she may be vulnerable, but she has to be strong, she has to be intelligent. She has to be independent and so does he, or I'm not interested in telling their stories," Nora says in a *Publishers Weekly* article.

Roberts has no patience for people who don't respect the romance genre. Her success has come almost completely without the recognition or respect of the mainstream media. In fact, her first *New York Times* book review (which she described as rather "snarky") ran in 2004—after she had already made their best seller list 125 times! In fact, *every* Nora Roberts book published since 1999 has made the *New York Times* list. According to Nora, "The romance novel at its core celebrates that rush of emotions you have when you are falling in love, and it's a lovely thing to relive those feelings through a book." Millions of women agree and over 250 million copies of her books are in print. That's about one for every man, woman, and child in America.

An avid reader, Roberts met her second husband when she hired him to build some bookshelves in her home. Talk about the beginning of a romance novel . . . She and her husband own a bookstore called Turn the Page in their hometown, which she credits with giving her plenty of access to books for research material, and keeps her in touch with her readers. Because she grew up surrounded by men—she was the youngest of five children, all the others being boys—she decided she had a choice between "figuring men out or running away screaming," according to her official website, noraroberts.com. Fortunately for us, she figured men out, and writes about them with humor, compassion and lusty appreciation.

"I started writing as a way to save my sanity," she said, "and I fell into a job I love."

CHAPTER 23

Be Your Own Heroine

Going on your own heroic journey will bring you pleasure

BUILDING A BRIDGE TO OUR FUTURE—MARIA

I am grateful and thankful to all the suffragettes, feminists, and women's rights activists who have worked for our freedom. Truly, I am. Each did the best that she could do. We would not be where we are today or have the freedom, choices, and options we do if those women hadn't suffered and worked hard for our good.

But somewhere, something went wrong. I know lots of women (even myself many, many years ago) who would say things like "I want to work and I believe in equality, but I'm *not* a feminist." The stereotype of a feminist, often fostered by conservative men, but sometimes confirmed by our own experiences, is that she is a bitter, angry woman who is a lesbian, or dresses like one. Feminism has been made a fringe movement. And while I'd like to say it's all men's fault, that would be perpetuating the problem.

I believe it's time to create a new ideal of feminine empowerment and freedom. Maybe it's even time to create a new word. To me, the key to creating a new future for women lies in building a bridge between all the feminists in the world and all the women who read romances. Can you imagine how big a bridge that would be? How powerful and strong women could be if we joined forces?

For centuries, writing was the only *legitimate* way for women to support themselves throughout history. From Christine De Pizan in the Middle Ages to the women of the 1800s who infuriated Nathaniel Hawthorne because their books outsold his (Maria Cummins's book *The Lamplighter* "sold four times as many copies in the first month as *The Scarlet Letter* sold in Hawthorne's lifetime." wrote Gail Collins in *America's Women*) to Nora Roberts today, women writing everything from Gothic romances to penny dreadfuls or today's chick lit have been quietly, diligently, prolifically supporting themselves, pleasing women everywhere, and creating an ever-changing ideal of female empowerment.

Many women who call themselves feminists have never read a romance because they automatically assume that it reinforces a stereotype of female submission. Not true. A romance heroine is really a feminist in a (sometimes) pretty dress, who loves men (eventually). A heroine is never quite done saving the world and making it a better place. She fundamentally believes that until all women are free and well-pleasured, until every child is loved and educated and every animal is treated with care and respect, and until every man is healed from his ancient wounds (caused by parents and society expecting him to be tough and violent), we are not done. Romance authors have been reinventing woman into heroic, *über*-powered Goddesses.

The romance heroine believes that women are inherently beautiful and strong and can achieve anything they set out to achieve, either in a corset and gown, a miniskirt, or a cowboy hat. She is not opposed to dressing like a man if her goal is to sneak into a gentleman's only club or ride a horse astride or escape a dangerous situation.

Romance heroines believe family is precious, but it doesn't define you. Having kids is wonderful and gives you the power of creating the next generation. But heroines also know that doing what they love makes them better mothers. You can succeed. You can run a business. You can have it all and be a great mom. You just have to do it differently, that's all. Some professional women have chosen not to have kids because they love their careers, or feel that having kids will hold them back. There is nothing wrong with that. Thanks to feminists they can make that choice. But some women are confused about their options. After I gave a speech at Columbia Graduate School of Journalism about launching a magazine, some of the young women came up to me and asked if I thought they could have children and still be successful in magazine publishing. "Other women—other top women magazine editors, even some who have kids—have told us we have to choose between motherhood and a career," they said. At the time I had a twenty-year-old and a five-year-old. "Ladies," I told them. "You *don't* have to choose between them. And having children is one of the most fulfilling things you can ever do. Do whatever makes you happy!"

Romance heroines believe that sex is amazing. At first they might be afraid of sex, or disappointed in prior experiences, but by finding their true love, they unleash their inner passion and learn the meaning of true pleasure. Sex is fun. Sex puts you in a good mood. Sex tames the "shrew" in all of us. And the hero *loves* the woman's body—every inch of it—and knows how to give her pleasure. He *enjoys* giving her pleasure. Neither feels shame about sexuality.

Romance heroines also know that our heroes need to be rescued, too. They need *us* to heal the pain they have been caused by being forced to grow up into "perfect" men. They need us to heal the emptiness they feel in their own souls. They need us to calm their own fears. Ultimately, men and women, heroes and heroines, need each other. That's a beautiful, beautiful thing.

I'm proud to call myself a feminist. I'm also proud to call myself a romance novel reader (but please, drop the "bodice-ripper" label). I don't want to be called a suffragette. It sounds too much like suffering. Instead, how about calling me . . . a pleasure revolutionary? Meanwhile, we would like to encourage any woman who calls herself a feminist to read romances, and support the *other* industry that has supported women with dignity for hundreds of years.

And romance readers, it's time to come out of the closet. Be proud of your passion and your strength. We are a huge and powerful group. Together, we are unstoppable.

HOW TO BE A HEROINE—MAYA

Sometimes we long to be the girl in the fairy tale, romance novel, or romantic comedy. I think we tend to fall in love with the hero

Develop your intuition, which is a fast-working kind of smarts. If he smells like a bad guy, he probably is. Our intuition is there to *keep* us out of bad or dangerous situations; our smarts are there to *get* us out of them.

4. *Don't shy away from the challenge or the adventure.* In most romances, desperate times call for desperate measures. Adventures place seemingly insurmountable obstacles in your way. This is the time to take chances, and act more daring than you thought you could.

5. *Run away, or rather, run towards something.* Nothing good happens to Cinderella until she gets out of the house. Same with Belle and the Beast. Same with any romance novel character. We all have dreams, fantasies, desires, and hopes. As a new heroine, go after them.

6. *Be open to falling in love.* A heroine has a good sense of who she is, and the confidence to be who she is. But she is not so stuck in herself that she can't recognize true love when it sweeps her off her feet (although sometimes it does take a few hundred pages for her to get there). A heroine finds real love with a man who doesn't try to compromise her, who doesn't demand she be someone she isn't. He doesn't love her for titles, money, or big breasts. Often, he loves her for the very same reasons others may ridicule her. He loves her for who she is.

7. *Never give up hope for happily ever after, and don't settle for less.* Who wants to read a story where the girl goes out, conquers all, and then settles for anything less than she deserves? Not me.

DO IT: HAVE A ROMANCE NOVEL WEEKEND

If you have never read romances, set aside a weekend and do it. There are so many different genres that one is guaranteed to appeal to you, whether it's hot contemporary, steamy historical, tough-action Western, sweet Christian inspirational, or time-travel fantasy. If you are too embarrassed to buy one at your local bookstore, supermarket, or warehouse price club, Amazon.com is a fabulous source of romance novels. Plus, you can read reviews the book has gotten and other readers' reviews and opinions to help you choose. (But don't be embarrassed—be proud! You are trying something new; you're going on an adventure!)

because really we just want to be the hero ourselves. If you want to l
heroine, you have to be tough, yet open to falling in love.

The heroines of our favorite stories are stubborn. They know wl
they want, and they don't let fools and villains stand in their way. Th
are smart, usually beautiful, but not always. Yet, they've got a spark th;
others simply cannot resist. They also love others and want to be loved
Sometimes their lives are hard. They may be orphans, or abused by evi
stepmothers and controlling fathers, but they never give up, and they
never let their troubles get them down.

Heroines take chances. Belle sees through the beast on the outside.
The princess kisses that squirmy frog. Cinderella goes out to the ball.
Women in romance novels are constantly turning down marriage proposals from men who are simply not The One. They run away from
lives that are unsatisfying and toward the lives they want. They take
chances and they are rewarded for it.

How can we be heroines in our own lives? You may not have actual
dragons to slay, or princes disguised as beasts, or threatening pirates,
but you can still find ways to be the heroine.

1. *Believe in yourself.* Because sometimes, no one else will. But if
you believe in yourself, like a heroine in her happy ending, you may
just get what you want, and what you deserve. And eventually, others
will have no choice but to say, "Wow. She's amazing." But you knew
you were all along.

2. *Get over the bad stuff.* I cannot think of one romance story in
which a heroine moped and sulked and cursed her situation. Such a
story would be too boring to tell. We all have tough circumstances in
our own lives, bad moods, or people who just want to bring us down. If
you want to be a heroine, you have to get over it. The girls from the
old stories didn't have therapy or twelve-step programs. These programs of course help countless numbers of people, but it is important
that you *not* spend your whole life revisiting old problems, moaning
about them and listening to others moan about theirs. Refuse to be a
victim.

3. *Get smart.* This includes street smarts, book smarts, and any
other smarts you need. Learn how to interpret nonverbal cues, or the
meaning behind the words, and communicate your desires and needs.
A true heroine can talk her way into or out of almost any situation.

Here are a few tips for making your weekend more than just a reading feast.

1. *Dress the part.* You don't have to do the full costume, but pay more attention than usual to dressing pretty and sexy so that you *feel* pretty and sexy. Dress like your favorite character in the book, or in another book you've read. You don't have to go outside your home so that people see you dressed up, just wander around your home in character.

2. *Do something daring.* Go for a horseback ride. Visit someplace you have never gone before. Explore something related to the topic of the book you're reading—like a museum or a location to see how the country or city looked in the book's time period.

3. *Be the heroine.* Imagine that you are as beautiful and desired as your heroine. It's amazing how much you start to feel like one!

LIST: OUR FAVORITE ROMANCE READING LIST— RATED PG (PLEASURE GUARANTEED)

Julia Quinn. Start with *The Duke and I.* Welcome to the Bridgerton Family. The mystery of just who the heck is Lady Whistledown goes on for a lot more books. They are so delicious!

Brenda Joyce. If steamy sex and complicated plots are your thing, Joyce is the best. A good one to start with is *After Innocence.* (We're not as taken with her stories set in contemporary times, but her historical novels are great.)

Emma Holly. Emma writes everything from historical to chick lit to vampire to hard-core erotica. Pick your fave.

Katherine Sutcliffe. The first one I picked up wasn't a historical—but I read it, and, as always, her heroines are tough, sexy, and strong. Good fun.

Lisa Kleypas. Lisa excels at the low-born heroes who make it big and the interesting heroines who unexpectedly fall in love with them. And the stories are loaded with hot sex.

Kathleen Woodiwiss. She's the woman who exploded the romance genre in America. Her epics are amazing. Her heroes are intense and her stories, while slightly dated (there are some rape scenes), are memorable. Maria's favorite: *Shanna*. Maya's favorite: *The Flame and the Flower*.

Georgette Heyer. Ruth Reichl read Heyer voraciously as a teen. The stories are very funny and truly British. Her work is a veritable fount of fantastic words due for a comeback.

Nora Roberts. You simply have to read one Nora Roberts novel if you want to understand what women want. She is the most-read author of anything. Her voice is smart-ass, tough, and no-nonsense. Her stories tend to be violent and bloody, but real page-turners.

Joan Johnston. Her Texas series spans generations—from the first settlers to modern times, with a good strong dose of Western spirit.

Eloisa James. She's a Shakspearean professor by day, a romance writer by night. She writes laugh-out-loud, cry-real-tears historicals that are pure pleasure.

IN HER OWN VOICE: ELIZABETH CADY STANTON

"Women have crucified the Mary Wollstonecrafts, the Fanny Wrights, and the George Sands of all ages. Men mock us with the fact and say we are ever cruel to each other . . . Let us end this ignoble record and henceforth stand by womanhood. If Victoria Woodhull must be crucified, let men drive the spikes and plait the crown of thorns."

"I think if women would indulge more freely in vituperation, they would enjoy ten times the health they do. It seems to me they are suffering from repression."

"I asked them why one read in the synagogue service every week the 'I thank thee, O Lord, that I was not born a woman.' 'It is not meant in an unfriendly spirit, and it is not intended to degrade or humiliate women.' But it does, nevertheless. Suppose the service read, 'I thank thee, O Lord, that I was not born a jackass.' Could that be twisted in any way into a compliment to the jackass?"

"So long as woman accepts the position that they assign her, her emancipation is impossible."

PLEASURE REVOLUTIONARY: ELIZABETH CADYSTANTON—
THE WOMAN WHO DOES IT ALL AND HAS IT ALL

Elizabeth Cady Stanton, veteran of women's suffrage, is the icon we've been missing, the real-life heroine, the woman who does it all. Stanton was an early pleasure revolutionary who believed that "self-development is a higher duty than self-sacrifice."

Born in 1815 in upstate New York, she got married and had a lot of kids. Interestingly, not many biographies dwell on this portion of her life, although we assume that it laid the foundation for her later work— giving birth to the women's movement. Stanton organized the famous Seneca Falls convention in 1848, where she called for the right of women to vote. She also rewrote the Declaration of Independence to include women as citizens and criticized the Bible as being the source of Western women's subjugation. And she did this all while being a devoted wife and mother.

Today, Stanton is primarily remembered for her part in the fight for women's right to vote, but she was really out to transform the entire world.

Her passion for activism started in 1840 at an abolitionist convention that she attended with her husband in London. There she met other women like herself who wanted to address the convention, but were forbidden and had to sit behind a screen and listen. That circle of women discovered their own oppression, which ran so deep that they could not even advocate others' freedom. Could this have been the beginning of men's uneasiness when women go to the ladies room in groups? What are they talking about in there? Are they planning some kind of revolution? Yes, oh yeah, definitely.

After London, Elizabeth and her friends organized the Seneca Falls convention, which called out to the world that something new, something big was starting. But on the carriage ride to the convention, Lucretia Mott and Stanton's husband begged Elizabeth not to demand the right to vote. When she did so anyway, her father, a physician, was called in to check her mental stability. In Stanton's mind, if a woman had to pay taxes (which she did), she should be able to vote on how her tax dollars were spent. Stanton insisted that women be more than their husbands' playthings and servants.

At the convention, Stanton also argued that the Bible, the so-called "word of God," was the source of many of society's excuses and practices for perpetuating female oppression. She realized that to rectify this injustice, common laws had to be changed to give women the right to education, to earn a living, to own property, to have rights to her children and her own body.

Elizabeth and her friends founded the National Women Suffrage Association, which later merged with the American Women's Suffrage Association, of which Elizabeth became president. Some younger members disagreed with Elizabeth's opinions of the role of religion in their oppression, but Elizabeth didn't punk out; she held fast to her beliefs, another attribute that makes her a heroine.

Elizabeth's partner in the revolution was Susan B. Anthony, and they worked closely through the years, with Susan doing the organizing and Elizabeth doing the writing. Susan eventually got a coin with her face on it, but our Elizabeth has no such distinction. Perhaps Susan got more recognition because she was "safer"; she never married or had children; she opposed abortion. She also was able to travel more and, hence, became the poster girl for the movement. She may unwittingly have been the origin of the negative stereotype of the feminist movement—single, seemingly nonsexual, and devoted to her work above all. But it was Elizabeth Cady Stanton who succeeded in doing what so many women struggle with today. She is The Woman Who Does It All: wife, mother, lover, writer, activist, president of a massive organization, speaker, organizer—all while having a fondness for both pants and fancy dresses. Elizabeth knew how to be the heroine of her own life, and she became a heroine in ours in well.

CHAPTER 24

Think Pink

Pleasure enjoys the feminine

IT'S OK TO BE A WOMAN (PRIDE IN MY CHICKEN SOUP)—MARIA

The other day I was on the bus to New York City and coming down with a cold. I thought that I should call Lou to see if he could pull a chicken out of the freezer for me to make soup with, but then I forgot. By the time I got home that night I was exhausted and even sicker. But when I opened the refrigerator it was like a universal chorus of angels broke out singing. There was a huge, organic, fresh-killed chicken (already plucked) from my mother, who raises chickens. My apologies to vegetarians, but I was thrilled.

The next morning, I woke up still sniffling, and put on one of my vintage aprons (I have an apron and vintage tablecloth collection). I filled the giant pot with water, put in the chicken, added salt, and let it simmer all day long until the whole thing fell to pieces and made the absolute perfect, golden, flavor-packed broth.

I'm famous in my family for my chicken soup. My daughters love, love, love it, and, even though my husband is a vegetarian, he finishes what they don't eat. Even my babysitter has said I make the best broth ever (she thinks it's the organic chickens). All I know is it hits the spot . . . and the simpler I keep it the better.

It took me a long time to figure that out. When I first started making soup and following recipes I would add onions, carrots, celery, other veggies and herbs. I'd experiment with different techniques. But now I know that the simplicity of chicken, water, and salt cooked all day long does the trick. An organic, free-range chicken is essential for the best flavor. Think of it like this: Garbage (bad feed, antibiotics, dark, cramped living conditions, and stress) in = garbage out . . . Favor (fresh air, sunlight, organic grains and grasses, and a few insects for protein) in = flavor out.

Does my chicken soup make colds magically disappear? No. But it does make your nose run. And studies have shown that something in chicken soup does hasten the healing of colds. And it makes people happy. Making my chicken soup makes me feel like a woman, like a mom, and maybe even a grandmom. In the simple, feminine act of making good soup I feel my power—the power of my love. It's such a great feeling and I wouldn't trade it for the world. I enjoy the feeling of business successes—of giving a good speech, getting media attention for our worthy causes. I don't want to stop doing all that. But in order to keep enjoying my work and business life, I *need* to keep making chicken soup and grounding myself in the primal, female world of home and love.

My chicken soup has been a constant in my life, but in other ways, I'm still in the process of reconnecting with my own femininity. I went through a serious phase while I was working my way up in the man's world where I wanted to hide and disguise my femininity. I did it in a number of ways: gained a lot of weight, wore baggy clothes, wore lots of black and gray, tried not to ornament myself with jewelry too much. I felt that I wanted to guard my sexuality from the men at work. I didn't want them to be attracted to me in any way other than for my fine mind.

During the worst days of the management changes I read tons of romances to survive, but the ones I loved most then I almost can't bear to read now. Back then I was into the war romances, in which a girl has to protect her castle from marauding barbarians and knows how to fight like hell and better than the men around her. In others, she has been exiled and is fighting her way back (usually dressed like a man). In still others, she's a war doctor or nurse tending to the wounded and falling in love while serving as a secret spy.

As things started to improve at work I read the more lighthearted, Regency-era stories of ballgowns and rakes. I started wanting to wear a corset. In 2001, I even walked into Bergdorf Goodman and asked if they carried any corsets. They looked at me as if I were daft, but two years later the corset was ubiquitous. Meanwhile, I noticed that most women where I come from in Pennsylvania have now moved to sexless clothing. It's less about the suit and more about the jeans, T-shirt, and sweatshirt. And they have short hair.

Lately I've lost ten pounds, thanks to the South Beach Diet, and I've been dressing a bit more womanly. I've got a curvy little body with boobs that don't need a pushup bra, but I still find it hard to find clothes that are feminine, not slutty, romantic but not tacky. I always joke with Maya that when I was her age and her size, I couldn't afford all the designer clothes. Now that I can afford them, not only can I barely fit in them, but I wouldn't be caught dead in most of them. I think the way women's magazines portray women in fashion shoots—they look dead, drugged, depressed, or totally empty—is repulsive. As Steve Murphy, our women-respecting CEO, says, "It's misogynistic." I have tried to change that portrayal with *Organic Style Magazine*.

After this fashion tirade is over, I'm going to put on a pretty dress and go make some chicken soup (without noodles . . . too many carbs).

THE RECIPE FOR CHICKEN SOUP: Take one whole or cut-up raw organic chicken. Cover it with water. Add a few teaspoons of salt. Bring to a boil. Skim the gunk off. Turn it down to simmer until the chicken falls to pieces and the stock is nice and golden (minimum of two hours, but four is good). Strain the broth. Add more salt to taste. By hand, pick out the good chicken meat and add back to the broth (or put aside for sandwiches).

LIVING THE BARBIE LIFE—MAYA

Oh, joy and rapture, I can still see it now: the hot pink glow of the Barbie aisle in the toy store. The pinkness softens the glare of fluorescent lights, the pink promise of many happy hours playing and pretending. The pink whispers a refuge for girls, a surrounding pink that feels almost womb-like. Heaven must be a similar pink.

One of my favorite childhood memories is sitting in my cousin's basement surrounded by girls and three generations of Barbie clothes and props, dresses my mom and her sisters sewed when they were kids and passed on to their daughters. My Aunt Heather handed down plastic Barbie kitchen appliances. An older girl we knew donated a two-story Barbie house. We built other houses out of blocks and videos. The clothes! The shoes! The Barbies with unfortunate haircuts from the days we decided to be hair stylists. We were deeply involved in our playing, so deep that my cousin even answered the phone in her "Barbie" voice—high and wispy—and we all dissolved into giggles. The hours, days, and months sitting with my cousins just playing and pretending is a shared memory and bond that will never go away.

Barbie has gotten a bad reputation these days, blamed for girls' insecurities with their bodies, eating disorders, plastic surgery, and unrealistic expectations. I think it's ridiculous to blame a seven-inch plastic doll. When you're a girl, Barbie, or any doll you have, is the one thing *you* are in charge of. Your dolls need you for life the way a child needs his or her mother. These dolls can live out the fantasies that, at a young age, you aren't allowed to pursue. My Barbies went on dates, had jobs and relationships. Playing with Barbie, imagining the life she had, was really my practice for being a well-adjusted grown-up. I have never heard of a girl who played "my Barbie has an eating disorder, is unhappy with her life, and is in an unfulfilling relationship with Ken."

In high school, a teacher of mine complained about his daughter playing with Barbies—"she just changes their clothes over and over," he said. "That's all that you see her doing," I replied. But her Barbie was changing out of her work clothes and into her workout clothes. Her Barbie had dates, got married, went to a friend's wedding, studied for a college exam. My Barbie even won the Miss America pageant we held in the basement. We like to marvel at children's imaginations—at the games they invent, when they go camping in forts made out of blankets and pillows from the couch, when they play house, when boys play war. But for some reason, Barbies are seen as psychological poison.

I think it is dangerous and irresponsible to condemn Barbie dolls. Little girls are sensitive to the things they hear. If grown-ups say a girl's favorite toy is a devil in disguise, and that playing with it will prepare her for a life of self-loathing, she may actually hear that imagining the life she wants to live is the key to unhappiness. In my family, playing with

Barbies was a celebrated tradition. I don't think a single female member of my family has suffered because of playing pretend with a plastic doll.

My basement play dates with my Barbies still live in my head. The lives my Barbies enjoyed stay with me. I am happy when I can finally do the things my Barbies did, like drive, have jobs and boyfriends, and go to college. When my high-heeled foot presses down on the gas pedal, I haven't forgotten the Barbies who went before me.

Once, just because I could, I bought a pair of hot pink Prada stilettos—if ever a pair of Barbie shoes were made for a real woman, these are IT. I saw them in the store, I coveted, I tried them on, I saved my money, and I bought them. They are my tribute to Barbie, and to the life she lived in my head, which I can now do for real. And mine is a happy, satisfying life full of love and imagination, and yes, clothes and shoes.

DO IT: GIVE YOURSELF A GIRLIE DAY

A girlie day is how you define it. What makes you feel most like your youthful self when you had no responsibilities, no to-do lists, no job come Monday morning? Here are some of our suggestions:

Dress up. Wear frilly, feminine things that feel soft and make you feel like a girl. Put on pink, put on your jewels, do up your hair, and look your most beautiful best.

Hang out with some girlfriends. Go to brunch together. Lounge around your bedroom or apartment telling secrets and sharing gossip.

Go shopping. Don't go to the supermarket or the Walmart. Go fun places. Shop for pretty things, or sporty things. Choose something symbolic just for you as you start out on your own pleasure revolution.

Play. Go for a bike ride. A walk or run through the woods. Swim and float and watch the clouds sail by. Play kick ball with some kids.

Go to the movies in the middle of the day. Eat popcorn with butter. See a romantic comedy! Or snuggle up on your couch and watch old movies on your TV.

Bake or cook. Make something that takes all day and makes the house smell like home. Bread. Cake. Pot roast. Have girlfriends over to share it, or take extras to someone who needs it.

Do some crafts. Put together a photo album. Pull out the sewing machine and make new pillows for your couch. Paint something—an old piece of furniture or a picture. Make cards out of construction paper and Elmer's glue and send them to people. Won't they be surprised?

LIST: THE NATURAL TALENTS OF WOMEN, ACCORDING TO HELEN FISHER

We women know that we have special powers, but now scientists and anthropologists have determined just what we're especially, innately good at. We're not saying that women are better than men, or vice versa, or that certain skills are more valuable than others, but over the last million years or so, we've developed these unique talents:

Multitasking and web thinking. After much research into the development of the brain in men and women, anthropologist Helen Fisher describes the way the female brain works as web thinking. Studies show that, generally, the bridge between the left and right brain hemispheres is thicker in women than in men, meaning women's brain functions are more interconnected. This may play a part in the holistic approach women tend to take in interpreting situations and making decisions. Other studies have noted women are also better at tackling many things at once—multitasking. Think of the classic if clichéd image of a woman holding a baby, supervising other children, talking on the phone, and making dinner simultaneously.

Communication. Studies have shown that women excel at picking up nonverbal cues, at reading gestures and facial expressions. Theoretically, this means women have an increased understanding and sensitivity to people and their feelings, which is probably why mothers are so good at telling when their kids are lying. Men's lesser ability in this area may be why men think women are interested in them, even when women are giving unmistakable "don't talk to me" nonverbal signals.

Women also have a talent with words. Some anthropologists theorize that this is because, as humans evolved in hunter-gatherer societies, women were the ones who needed to communicate verbally—with other women, or their children—while the men needed to stay silent while hunting. Today, 54 percent of contemporary American book authors are women. Men tend to speak up more in social situations, but women tend to have in-depth conversations amongst themselves. Studies show that girl babies babble more than infant boys and generally outperform boys on aptitude tests measuring language abilities.

Empathy and nurturing. Centuries of mothering, working closely with other women in the home and communities, and our ability to understand nonverbal communication have helped women develop skills at empathizing and nurturing. But certain hormones also play a part. Estrogen, which is prominent in females, is "clearly associated with nurturing behavior in many mammalian species, including humans," says Helen Fisher. Oxytocin, which surges during the birthing process and after a woman has an orgasm, has been nicknamed the "cuddle hormone" because it promotes affectionate and nurturing behavior.

Long-term strategic thinking. Whether investing in the future financially or biologically, women more than men tend to plan long-term, which is done in the prefrontal cortex, also the impulse-control center. Men's and women's prefrontal cortexes are different in structure, so it is quite possible that women's brains are wired for long-term strategic thinking.

IN HER OWN VOICE: ELOISE

"I holed in at the Plaza and we went to work. I just knew I had to get this done. Eloise was trying to get out. I've never known such stimulation. This girl had complete control of me. Ideas came from everywhere. Hilary and I had immediate understanding. . . . We wrote, edited, laughed, outlined, cut, pasted, laughed again, read out loud, laughed and suddenly we had a book."

KAY THOMPSON, AUTHOR OF THE *ELOISE* BOOKS

"I love love and I believe in divorce. Two great things. I've lived with quite a few men and alone is better. That doesn't mean I'm a loner; I just don't like to ask permission."

KAY THOMPSON

"I am Eloise
I am six
I am a city child
I live at The Plaza"

"ooooooooo I absolutely love Room Service
they always know its me
and they say "Yes Eloise?"
and I always say "Hello, this is me ELOISE and would you
kindly send one roast-beef bone, one raisin and seven spoons
to the top floor and charge it please
thank you very much"

"then I hang up and look at the ceiling
for a while and think of a
way to get a present"

PLEASURE REVOLUTIONARY: KAY THOMPSON, AUTHOR OF *ELOISE*—GRACE, ELEGANCE, AND PIZAZZ

Kay Thompson was born Kitty Fink and grew up to invent and embody pizazz, the American version of *je ne sais quoi*. She was a singer, actress, dancer, fashion designer, and, most famously, the mother and inventor of the beloved, perpetually age-six troublemaker, Eloise.

She grew up in St. Louis, Missouri, but details of Thompson's childhood are few because of her reluctance to discuss it. Quite the piano prodigy, she played with the St. Louis Symphony at the age of fourteen, reportedly tripping over a potted plant on her way off stage. She described herself as "a stage struck kid," and at seventeen skipped town to be a radio vocalist. After her show flopped, she said, "I came to a serious decision. I had to be an actress and I had to be alone. So I went to Hollywood where I was neither."

Kay started working at MGM and became successful arranging and composing songs. Frank Sinatra said she taught him everything he knew about singing; she coached Judy Garland and the two later struck up a friendship. Kay was Liza Minnelli's godmother. After a few years, her contract with the studio up, Kay put together a nightclub act, which became an enormous success, featuring "sophisticated songs" sung by Kay and backed by the four Williams Brothers. As a group they started off earning $2,500 a week, but were soon earning $15,000 a week. One reviewer wrote, "Miss Thompson is more than an act, she's an experience."

Eloise was conceived on tour. When the perpetually punctual Kay just happened to be late one day, she offered her excuse in a wispy voice, saying, "I am Eloise. I am six." As her six-year-old alter ego, Kay came up with outrageous stories to entertain her group on the road.

After six years, the tour was over, and Kay took time off to decorate her Beverly Hills home and design a line of trousers called "Kay Thompson's fancy pants." She concocted another show, in which she portrayed a blasé hostess entertaining imaginary guests on stage. Kay got a gig at the Persian Room in the Plaza Hotel, and free accommodations at the hotel, where she stayed for many years (until Donald Trump's management kicked her out). Friends who adored the playful character of Eloise encouraged Kay to write a book. In 1954 she met illustrator Hilary Knight through a mutual friend and gave him twelve lines in "Eloisian." A few months later she received a Christmas card from him, showing Eloise hitching a ride on Santa's sleigh. Soon after, the two were holed up at the Plaza, giving birth to Eloise. The book debuted in November 1955 and was an instant success.

Eloise was more than just a commercial success. The first book's subtitle was "for precocious adults," but Eloise struck a nerve with women and girls of all ages. With her unsupervised freedom at the Plaza, she doesn't have to go to school, her mother is mysteriously absent, and her nanny devoted. She has a two-page, illustrated temper tantrum, talks on paper cups to Mars, goes to grown-up parties uninvited and unchaperoned, calls room service whenever she wants and orders whatever she wants with a "thank you very much and charge it please!" She's wildly imaginative, flip, and just plain *fun*. Apparently, Eloise is a lot like Kay Thompson herself.

In 1957, taking a break from Eloise, Kay landed the role of a fashion magazine editor in the Audrey Hepburn classic *Funny Face*. She opens the movie with a song and dance called "Think Pink!" She didn't think her diversity of talents was unusual at all: "If artistically you are able to do one thing, you are more likely to do them all."

Kay stood five feet, five inches, but seemed to be seven feet tall. She was incredibly stylish, witty, funny, and dramatic. When questioned about her habit of feeding her darling pug a diet of lime chuckles and chocolate covered cherries, "she would declare 'the drapes are on fire' and leave the room." As her goddaughter, Liza Minnelli, said, "Once upon a time there was this amazing woman who could do anything, and once you saw her do it, it was too late to analyze what it was she did because she had already changed your life forever."

Kay died in 1998. She left behind Eloise, unpublished works, forty pairs of shoes, confusion about her real age, and the devilishly brilliant idea to pour water down the mail chute.

vn hero helps me be a heroine

nce novels and from life: True
be your true self (and vice-versa).

TIC COMEDY—MAYA

ith romantic comedies; they are my
l, my source of tears of joy. I have
of mine, but I don't mind, because I
love being resolved happily in two
short stories in which the formula of a
ass, and I see every little love affair,
ced in its terms.
ork, I was smarting and separated from a
was at large in the city. I wrote an epic
fe Were a Romantic Comedy." I invented
andomly on the street, scripting them as
ovie screen. For example, I imagined turn-
ashington Square Park, walking smack into
where, and then there would be a dramatic
think of something to say.
nvolved with this story, the more I came to real-
ore going on in every romantic comedy (at least,
ve story between "just a girl, standing in front of a
otting Hill). Romantic comedy heroes are often the
e different from romance novel heroes who are the
a romantic comedy any boy and any girl can be the
in real life, translates to far more opportunities for
is also a "male foil" or "female foil"—someone who
on. In the movie *French Kiss*, the male foil is the fiancé
Ryan, and whom she spends most of the movie chasing
that he isn't The One at all. Chewing on a pencil as I
I wondered if the boy I was obsessing over was The
l. The question was answered when I got involved with
nd forgot about the story and its "hero."

a romantic comedy hero, but in a romance novel?!

CHAPTER 25

If Your Life Were a Novel

Pleasure wants you to create

your own story

MY LIFE, THE ROMANCE NOVEL—MARIA

I was on a trail ride through a beautiful old Pennsylvania forest on a crisp fall day with a hint of wood smoke, horse, and decaying leaves in the air. Lou and Eve were with me. I said to my lovely cowgirl riding teacher, who was leading the ride, that this was the perfect scene for pretending to be in a novel.

"Oh, I do that all the time," she said. "I love to shovel snow because I pretend that I'm in Russia and I have to shovel a path out to get food for my children." Ah, a girl after my own heart.

Historical romances are my favorite kind of romance novels. The contemporary ones are fine in a pinch, but to tell you the truth I find the insecurities of the chick lit heroine slightly boring (I'm over it) and the frequent materialism of the mainstream contemporary slightly empty. I already wear designer clothes if I feel like it, so I don't need to fantasize about it. Plus, I know what the limits are to the pleasure and happiness that those things bring (expensive shoes give you blisters just as easily as cheap shoes).

But give me a horse, a time when there were no phones, no electricity, no Internet and I am free, free, free. I relate best to the spunky, over-the-top historical heroines. I know that in real life they probably wouldn't have been that liberated and that adventurous—and they probably had hair under their armpits and on their legs—but I don't care. I used to think the heroes were probably physically unreali until I took to watching some of the PBS reality shows like "Frontic House," "Colonial House," and "Manor House," and my favorite, "Regency House Party." Before your eyes, modern men are transformed into the lean, strong romance heroes of yore from all the hard physical labor that daily life required and from the absence of all the carbs and conveniences of modern life that make us weaker and puffier (myself included). You can also see that yesterday or today, no man is a hero if he lacks honor and integrity. That's what really matters.

I don't stick with one time period or country but I like to pick and choose according to what I'm going through in my own life at the time. Sometimes at work I'm a character in the old war novels, trying to figure out ways to win a battle, understand the mind of "the villain," and protect my family. More often these days I'm a rodeo cowgirl in an old Western, trying to stay on a bucking bull or rope an ornery calf. When I'm working in New York I'm really in the London *"ton"* of 1820, dealing with rakes, dandies, society snobs, and mean gossips, wishing people still traveled by horse and coach instead of bus or taxi.

When I was doing research for this book and writing, I often pretended that I was in the Middle Ages or even earlier, secretly trying to uncover our feminine history. I know if I am discovered I would be tried for witchcraft or burnt as a heretic. Whenever I would take a break, I would be very thankful to be living today, because it wasn't too long ago that this book would have been considered heresy. In some circles, it still is.

I'm not looking for my hero, anymore. I've got one. The longer I've been married (twelve years), the more Lou has become my hero. He not only puts up with all my crazy notions and hoydenish behavior, but seems to love me for it. He is always there for me when I need him—with a strong hand or a wise, kind word. He definitely has the honor and integrity of a hero, and he never treats me poorly. I am impressed by the genuineness of his spiritual faith, and his tolerance of my different opinions. Oh, he's got his flaws (we all do), but they are small compared to his strengths, and those flaws actually help me

akimbo, and dealing with it. And my ov
through it all.

Here's what I learned from roma
love is finding someone who lets you

MY LIFE, THE ROMAN

You could say I am obsessed w
frame of reference, my ide
endured ridicule about this love
understand the gloriousness of
hours. I also love writing many
romantic comedy is my com
crush, or fling I have experien
When I moved to New Y
former flame. He, like me,
short story, called "If My Li
scenarios of us meeting r
they would happen on a m
ing the corner around W
him, papers flying every
pause as we each tried t
The more I became
ize that there was far m
the good ones) than a l
boy" (Julia Roberts, N
boy next door. They'
masculine ideal.* In
leading stars, which
love. Usually, there
serves as a distract
who ditched Meg
until she realizes
wrote my stor
One, or The
a different

T
have
for in
music,
more. O
to write th
and I are bu
historical hon

A romance
optimism and o
overcome any crisi
eration for cancer, l
times before—in the
face any danger and co
in love . . . with my her
letting life happen to me.
Sure, there are surprises—t
are tragedies—that's life. But
ness. I'm facing them and all

* Billy C

With the second boy, I continued to pretend we were acting out the script of a romantic comedy. I saw myself as the slightly awkward but ultimately lovable leading actress. I wrote another short story. Writing satisfied the need for therapy. In real life, I kept waiting for the second boy to come to the conclusion I had already reached: that he needed to love me so we could be happy together. I tried something that always works in the movies—the dramatic, deeply honest confession of love. It didn't translate well from the silver screen—in fact, it was an utter failure, and we never spoke again. That put me in a state of emotional despair. This was not the movie I signed on for! I became cynical, as many romantic comedy heroines do at some point in the plot. I wrote a bitter conclusion to my second short story: I forget that I am a real girl in a real world. And reality is the only bastard in the world who never fails to show up, who calls when he says he will, who will be there for you on your birthday, who will sit with you while you cry, who will have breakfast with you on Sunday mornings. Too bad I don't find him more attractive.

But I was reaching the absolutely pivotal moment of a revelation in a romantic comedy. A shining example of it is in the Ashley Judd film *Someone Like You:* broken-hearted, she finds herself saying about her ex,* "He is not the only man I ever loved, or the only man that will ever love me." At that moment, she realizes the man she thought was The One was actually The Foil. But you can see in her face that she also realizes that she loves herself, she deserves real love, and she knows just where to get it. In romantic comedies, the revelatory moment happens immediately before the Mad Dash. The hero or heroine frantically runs through the streets of New York or some other big city, stopping traffic and knocking over fellow pedestrians, hair flying in the wind, a speeding car driven by the heart.

Real life often doesn't have such a neat, clear conclusion. So, for a while, I put "If My Life Were a Romantic Comedy" on the shelf. The essential next scene that usually moved the plot forward—the meeting—just didn't happen. The customary separation is essential for soul-searching and an eventual reunion of the lovers. Except we stayed separated.

I did have my moment, months later. I was relaxing in Washington

* Considered suing for breach of contract.

Square Park. And there he was, walking past, too fast for me to catch up, since I was wearing high heels. He was too far away to hear if I yelled. I stood up, calculating how I could catch up and make it look nonchalant. This was my moment, I realized. Should I go? Should I stay? The moment was loaded, hugely metaphorical, bigger than life size, made for the big screen.

I made a halfhearted effort to follow him. By the time I reached the corner of Waverly and University Place he had crossed, and the light had changed. If my life were a romantic comedy, I would have done the Mad Dash, and narrowly escaped being run over by a taxi. I would have shouted his name, and he would have turned, and there I would have been, The Girl. We would've embraced and had a happy ending. But I stood on the corner, debating. The sign said Don't Walk. So I crossed the street in the other direction and walked away.

But a year or two later I did find a different sort of happy ending. One day, after my boyfriend—who was not either of the Foils mentioned above—and I had been together for about a year, I was looking over my old stories, and came to a realization: My boyfriend has never failed to show up, he calls when he says he will, he's there for me on my birthday, sits with me while I cry, and has breakfasts with me on Sunday mornings.

DO IT: WRITE OUT THE STORY OF YOUR LIFE

Start with "once upon a time" and go from there. Go ahead, dramatize it and have fun. Make the villains truly awful. Make the heroes truly heroic. But most of all, put yourself in the center of the action and decide how you want it to evolve. Refer to positive stories you love to give you ideas. Don't use horror stories and tragedies. You want your life to go well. Watch some of our suggested Pleasure Revolution movies and read some of our favorite romances to give yourself some good ideas.

Remember, you are the author of your own life story. And you are the heroine. Saving the day is up to you. It's all in your hands.

LIST: THE PLEASURE REVOLUTION MOVIE LIST

There are so many great movies—some of which were shown only in art-house theatres—that are full of pleasure. When the credits roll, you can't help but feel happy and full, feeling the power of pleasure. If you need a jolt of pleasure, these movies will do the trick.

Babette's Feast. A woman transforms a whole town with one delicious meal.

Strictly Ballroom. A man and a woman bring new steps and new life to dance.

The Sound of Music. For utter joy go see the big screen sing-along version.

Enchanted April. Rediscovering pleasure in the Italian Riviera.

Orlando. The best thing to come out of Virginia Woolf ever.

Paperback Romance. An Aussie love story filled with laughter.

The Princess Bride. So she's not the best Pleasure Revolutionary. Still it's wonderfully funny.

Roman Holiday. For the princess in all of us.

Pride and Prejudice. The long version with Colin Firth is worth every minute.

Legally Blonde. Sheer pleasure!

IN HER OWN VOICE: GEORGE SAND

"Life is a novel that each of us carries within us."

"That women differ from men, that heart and intellect are subject to the laws of sex, I do not doubt. . . . But ought this difference, so essential to the general harmony of things, to constitute a moral inferiority?"

"Charity toward others;
Dignity toward oneself;
Sincerity before God."

"There is nothing strong in me except the need to love."

"I will lift women up from their abject state, both in my life and in my writings."

"We will love, we will suffer, we will hope, we will be afraid, we will be full of joy, of terrors, in a word we will go on living, because life is like that, a terrible mix. Let us love and support each other."

PLEASURE REVOLUTIONARY: GEORGE SAND

A complicated woman—famous and infamous, loathed and loved, notorious and yet now almost forgotten—George Sand was alive when few women or men dared to live in a way that would cause scandal. But nothing, and no one, stopped her from living dramatically and romantically.

Born Aurora Dupin in Paris, she was almost illegitimate. Her titled father had married her bohemian prostitute mother twenty-six days before her birth on July 5, 1804. Her parents had a passionate love match that ended when her father was thrown from a horse and killed when she was only five—only days after her baby brother had also died.

Her mother was slightly mad and unstable, yet brilliantly inspiring and loving. She left the five-year-old Aurora with her mother-in-law and returned to Paris from their country home, Nohant, to care for her children from a previous liaison. She realized her daughter would be better cared for and educated with her mother-in-law, but for Aurora, the separations and reunions followed by further separations were devastating. Like most of our early pleasure revolutionaries, Aurora received a "boys' education." When her grandmother died, she was sent back to Paris to live with her mother, who worried about Aurora's interest in books and her cool self-control.

In Aurora's late teens, she began dressing as a man in order to ride astride, but soon found she enjoyed the freedom and ability to experiment that it provided her. When she was eighteen, she married Casimir Dudevant, believing that their strong friendship would be the basis of a good marriage, but his unsentimental, unromantic nature proved difficult for Aurora to live with. She persevered and less than a year later gave birth to a son, Maurice, whom she breast-fed, which was very socially incorrect at the time. By the time she had been married eight years, both her husband and she were openly having affairs. A few years after Maurice was born, she gave birth to Solange, believed to be the daughter of a lover in Paris.

Aurora had a passion for writing and began to develop it as a potential means of financial independence, since her husband was squandering their resources. In 1830 she met Jules Sandeau, who became her lover when she was twenty-six and he nineteen. Shortly after, while looking for something in her husband's desk, she found a letter he had written to be opened on his death in which he spoke of his disgust for her. That was the catalyst she needed. She decided to move to Paris, leaving her young children behind at Nohant until she could figure out how to support them. Once again, she dressed as a man and soon realized that the only way to bring her children to Paris was to earn enough money as a writer. She became the only woman working on the staff of *Figaro*, got her own flat, and hosted salons with guests like Honoré de Balzac.

Jules Sandeau, still her lover, and she jointly published their first major article in 1831 and signed it J. Sand. She published her first novel, *Indiana*, under the pseudonym George Sand; since it was scandalous for a woman to make a living as a writer in those days, none of her relatives wanted their name associated with her writing. When *Indiana* first appeared in 1832, Balzac praised it, and most readers were enthusiastic about it, but critics hated it. Nonetheless, it became a commercial success and launched her prolific writing career. In one of the many introductions she later added to the book, she writes: "I wrote Indiana out of deep and genuine feelings . . . about the barbaric injustice of the laws that still control a woman's existence within marriage, family, and society. I was not interested in writing a treatise on law, but in waging war against public opinion, because that is what propels or postpones social change. The war will be a long and difficult one; but I am not the first, the only, or the last champion of such a noble cause, and I will fight for it as long as I have a breath of life."

In breaking the "rules" of good society by uncovering the misery of an awful marriage and giving the cheating heroine a happy ending, *Indiana* caused a scandal. Even Victor Hugo was upset. Jules was jealous, and they broke up. Afterwards, George may have had a lesbian affair with an actress. She wrote many more books. She took more lovers. She hung out with Franz Liszt. After a lot of nastiness, she finally got a divorce from Casimir and gained custody of her children.

In 1836 she met Frédéric Chopin. She was androgynous, leaning towards the masculine side. The composer was androgynous leaning towards the feminine. He was ill most of their long (for her) and peaceful (until the end) relationship and she mothered and protected him, which allowed him to create some of his best work. He wrote during the day. She wrote during the night. Today, George Sand is more renowned for her great affair with Chopin (and perhaps for dressing in men's clothing) than for any of her own writing, which is a shame. Her writing flies off the page and is filled with erotic intensity and sexual ambiguity, surprisingly readable and delightful.

To help Chopin's health, they went to Majorca. "That is where he composed the most beautiful of those brief pages that he modestly entitled Preludes," she writes in her memoir. "They are chef-d-oeuvres. Several bring to mind the visions of dead monks and echoes of funeral chants, which besieged him. Others are melancholy and sweet. These came to him during hours of sunlight and health, to the noise of the children's laughter beneath the window, the distant sound of guitars, the song of birds under the wet foliage, the sight of little pale roses blooming in the snow."

After eight years, Solange, her daughter, caused them to split. Solange had always had a very difficult relationship with her mother, and a very flirtatious relationship with Chopin. She chose to marry a sculptor, Jean-Baptiste Clesinger, which Chopin vehemently opposed, but Sand supported. After her marriage Solange discovered him to be massively in debt as well as abusive, and, after a violent incident in Sand's home, he was banished, along with Solange, by her mother. Chopin was so upset with George over Solange's marriage that he cut things off with her. Aside from a brief visit when Chopin coldly informed Sand that she had become a grandmother (the baby died a week later), they never saw each other again. He died later that year, and Sand, forty-five, was devastated.

Sand threw her energy into French politics. She even impressed Tocqueville, who had said of her before he met her "I detest women who write." After they met, he said "I like her." She wrote *The Story of My Life*, her autobiography, which was over a thousand pages long, then wrote twenty-four plays, of which six were very successful. Sand also settled into a loving, domestic long-term relationship with Alexandre Manceau. As Solange's marriage fell apart, her little daughter, Nini, went to live with George, providing her with some of her most happy days. But in a fit of paternal vengeance, Clesinger took her away and out into the chilly winter weather, after which Nini caught a fever and died at age five. Manceau died soon after of consumption.

George settled into a chaste domestic family life with her remaining grandchildren. She continued writing until the end, completing almost sixty novels. In 1876, she died of a stomach ailment. Her final words to her beloved grandchildren were "leave greenness . . ."

While she was alive, her influence was tremendous. In *A Writer's Notebook*, Dostoevsky wrote that, in spite of the ban on nonfiction, especially from France, in Russia during his youth, "The mass of readers in the 1840s, in our part of the world at least, knew that George Sand was one of the most brilliant, the most indomitable, and the most perfect champions." After her death, Sand's reputation suffered. Intellectual critics condemned her for her happy endings, and with the rise of Victorian (non)sexual values, her work went largely out of print and off the critically acclaimed reading lists.

Today, her reputation is ambiguous. In *A Song to Remember*, a movie about Chopin, made in 1944, Merle Oberon plays Sand as a domineering, bitter, stern, cross-dressing taskmaster. The 1990 film, *Impromptu*, with Hugh Grant as Chopin and Judy Davis playing Sand, portrays her as histrionic and out of control. In real life, Sand was neither histrionic nor domineering. She didn't want to be a man in the flawed social system of war and destruction, but she didn't want to be a woman who was held back by the strict rules of the day. In the end, Ivan Turgenev, the Russian writer, described her best: "What a brave man she was, and what a good woman."

CHAPTER 26

Love What You Do

Pleasure wants you to be happy

STUMBLING TOWARD ECSTASY
(FROM "CEO" TO WRITER)—MARIA

Why did my father pick me to succeed him? That question haunted me for years. In many ways I was not the obvious choice. I was not the oldest or the youngest. I was not male. I wasn't already a top executive, but a middling one. A few months before my father's death, Lou and I had been trying to figure out what we wanted to do with our lives—after all, we could really do anything we wanted. We were at the time seriously considering a move to New Zealand and were both excited by the idea. So I asked my father what his plans were. "I need to start planning my life," I said. We were in the kitchen of my parents' house in the middle of the day—which was where I found him more and more.

"I'm counting on you," he said.

"But it's such a burden," I replied, thinking of all the heavy responsibility.

"It's also a gift." He was wearing jeans, wool socks, and a flannel shirt, and was making a cup of tea.

I know I was supposed to be glad he was counting on me and a small part of me was. But a bigger part of me heard the metal doors clanking shut. There would be no New Zealand. My path was set. I had to stick around. Sure, I could have run off halfway across the world, anyway, but I think my father understood that I am responsible and honor my commitments. But I never, ever expected him to die so soon.

Right after he died, everyone just assumed (including myself) that I would one day become CEO and run the company. But in the secret velvet of my heart I didn't really want the job. In many ways I was very fortunate that he had designated my mother the interim chairwoman. It gave me time to find my footing and figure things out, which took a long time. About ten years.

There are parts of business I truly love. And now I understand what I am really good at—long-term strategy, identifying new markets and developing products for them. That hideously overused phrase, "thinking outside of the box," is, in fact, a specialty of mine. Because I love to read everything from history to science to celebrity gossip I have a unique ability to put disparate things together into interesting ideas and combinations. I'm not the greatest public speaker or the most organized executive, but the people who work with and for me seem to like me. I don't need them to like me, but it makes life more enjoyable.

Seven years after my father died we were working with a business consultant, and I was feeling pressure to step up and commit to being CEO. I was waffling and waffling. Then, one day, it hit me. I didn't have to be CEO. As an owner I could be vice-chairman, and eventually chairman, and I could hire good people who would *want* to be CEO. That would give me time to keep one Prada-clad foot in the business world so I wouldn't turn into a total reclusive crazy lady and the other foot snug inside my UGG boot. (I have to keep alternating feet to make sure one foot doesn't get jealous of the other.)

Since I made that decision—to move towards what I love and away from what I don't—everything fell into place. We have hired fantastic people who have hired even more fantastic people and business just booms. My family relationships improved. My relationship with my mother improved. I love my job so much more and I love writing even more, because I'm not conflicted about it. I know I love it and it knows I love it. I sleep really well at night.

We are all given a certain lot in life that is both a burden and a gift . . . the family, the place, the time we are born into. Everyone has some kind of inheritance. I've seen plenty of rich kids with a poverty of love, and poor kids with a wealth of love. All of our lots in life are both a burden and a gift. It's up to each of us to take the burden and turn it into a gift—honing it gently and persistently into something we love.

Maybe one day I will be CEO. If I need to I know I can. But I'll do it only if I really want to. If it feels right. I reserve the right to change my mind, to grow and evolve. But here's what I know for sure: When in doubt I'll always choose love.

YOU CAN'T QUIT THE PROCESS—MAYA

Sometimes I get everything I want and work for, and then I hate it. When the "be careful what you wish for" voice starts singing in my head, I want to punch it out. But I don't because of something Willy Wonka said: The only way out is through.

For example, after I had gotten a job and an internship at the same time, my weekly schedule went something like this for months without a single day off: back-to-back classes Monday and Wednesday; work Tuesday, Friday, Saturday, Sunday; internship Thursday and Friday. I inevitably got sick from overextending myself, eating poorly, and not taking time to rest. I was also taking time to go out with friends, which is when I came to the conclusion that you can't quit the process.

The process is figuring out how to live your life in a happy, balanced, satisfying way through trial and error. Even if you quit everything and move to a cabin in the woods, it's still part of the process. The process is not merely surviving, although that's certainly a part of it—it's dreaming and achieving and periodic deconstruction and reconstruction.

I had gotten what I wanted—a busy life. But then I found out it didn't fit quite right. So instead of making myself wear it, and making myself miserable, I changed the outfit. I simplified—stopped doing what I didn't like, and did more of what I did enjoy. I finished up the internship, and didn't get another one. I kept the job, and arranged my schedule so that even though I was busy, I at least had a day off. I shrugged and readjusted when the load became too heavy. The beauty of the periodic shrugs is that they shift the weight until it feels right. I graduated from college, I replaced the part-time job answering phones with a full-time job writing. The process can take years.

Even my dream job starts to hurt sometimes, specifically in my neck and shoulders. Sitting in a folding chair and typing day after day takes a toll physically and emotionally. When I caught myself complaining about my own pleasure revolution, rather than punk out—because pleasure revolutionaries do not punk out—I took a time-out.

I got out of the city and went off to a spa in the Berkshires alone, without a pen and paper or cell phone. As I drove on New England highways in autumn, enjoying fall foliage, singing along to musicals at the top of my lungs, I thought that this was what I needed. As I relaxed in the hot tub, got a massage, and lounged in the sauna I felt closer. I read a romance novel. I dined alone. I went on a bike ride and savored my solitude and silence. When all the kinks and pains were massaged and yoga-ed out of my body, I started to feel better. On my last night, while lying on the floor in a restorative yoga class, focusing on nothing but my breath, I heard the voice that said, "I want to go home." I missed my early morning writing sessions. I missed the way my keyboard started to squeak after a long day of typing. I missed being "engaged passionately with the world."

At the end of one of my favorite romantic comedies, *The Very Thought of You*, a character says that we make thousands of choices every day without thinking or agonizing about them. And just because we made a decision once doesn't mean it's carved in stone forever. We constantly choose the path we're on and the way we live. We remake those choices every single day. To make your choice with assurance, sometimes you have to take time out in order to figure out what you really need and really want. That's the pleasure way.

DO IT: MAKE A LIST OF ALL THAT YOU LOVE. NOW MAKE IT YOUR JOB

This one is easy. Take a clean tablet and make a list. Put down all the things you love most . . . people, activities, places, hobbies, daily rituals, food.

Now look at your list and look at it good. If you had to create a job out of your list, what would it be? Sit with it a while. Take a shower (it's the source of so many good ideas). See what comes up.

You don't have to quit what you are doing tomorrow and do what's on your list right away. The first thing to notice is how close your real daily life is to what's on your list. The second thing is to think about what you can change to make it closer.

Who knows, you might just discover a whole new business, or uncover a long lost dream.

LIST: THE EVIDENCE—PLEASURE IS GOOD FOR YOU

(Notice that almost all these studies have been done on men, not women!)

Sex. Boosts your immune system, as long as you have it at least once or twice a week. Orgasms can even relieve headaches and menstrual cramps. No word on whether or not you need a partner in order to reap the benefits, although men who ejaculate at least three times a week (by any means) have 33 percent less of a chance of developing prostate cancer.

Chocolate. Dark chocolate is rich in antioxidants and flavonoids and improves your blood circulation. A Finnish study found that moms who eat chocolate during pregnancy (especially the ones who are feeling stressed) have happier babies!

Novelty. *The Journal of Neuroscience* reports that people get more pleasure out of the unexpected than the expected. Helen Fisher suggests doing new activities with a lover, as a way to keep the spark alive.

Hobbies. Kids who have hobbies and play sports do better at school and are better developed emotionally and behaviorally, according to a Penn State study. Knitting and embroidery can help arthritic hands. Losing yourself in a task—otherwise known as "flow"—is one of the keys to happiness, according to a University of Illinois study. Keeping your brain stimulated by taking classes and socializing keeps your brain young, according to a British study.

Friends. Having friends is just as important to overall health as diet and exercise. In fact, family, friends, meaningful activities, and the ability to forgive are all connected to feeling happy and living a long life.

Food. Americans have the most obsessive, guilt-ridden relationship with food of any nationality, and we are the fattest. Despite our low-fat,

low-carb, crazy food concerns, as Michael Pollan writes in a *New York Times* magazine article, "cultures that set their culinary course by the lights of pleasure and habit rather than nutritional science are actually healthier than we are, suffer a lower incidence of diet-related health troubles. Americans worry more about food and derive less pleasure from eating than people in any other nation they [U.S. and French academics] surveyed." Guilty feelings about food actually cause Americans to gorge more (and then feel even guiltier).

Vacations. A study of 12,338 men found that the more times they skip their annual vacation, the more likely they are to die. Don't take a chance—go without him.

In general, pleasurable effects last longer than negative stimuli, and not having enough pleasant experiences is a major stress on the immune system. A report in the *New York Times* states that doing without life's "little pleasures" made men more likely to get colds.

So America, *stop feeling guilty!*

IN HER OWN VOICE: JULIA QUINN

"'Men are sheep. Where one goes, the rest will soon follow.'
Lady Whistledown's Society Papers, 30 April 1813"
—*THE DUKE AND I*

"'Rosamund Reiling swears that she saw Benedict Bridgerton back in London. This Auithor is inclined to believe the veracity of the account; Miss Reiling can spot an unmarried bachelor at fifty paces.
Unfortunately for Miss Reiling, she can't seem to land one.'
Lady Whistledown's Society Papers, 12 May 1817
—*AN OFFER FROM A GENTLEMA*

"Dunford raised a brow. *This* was Henry? "You're a girl," he said, rea izing how stupid he sounded even as the words left his mouth.
"Last time I looked," she said cheekily . . .
Quite honestly, Dunford didn't want to get within three feet of h
Henry had been wearing eau de piglet since morning and h grown quite used to it."
—*M*

PLEASURE REVOLUTIONARY: JULIA QUINN—
THE HARVARD ROMANCE WRITER

Julia Quinn went to Harvard and dropped out of Yale medical school to write romances. She created the Bridgerton family, and the mysterious Lady Whistledown, who figure in a hysterical, historical, and delightful Regency world of romance. Julia has won numerous awards for her writing, and made it onto *The New York Times* best seller list a few times. So far, she has *only* written thirteen romances, but over 2.5 million of them are in print.

In her thirties with two children, Julia is married to a doctor who is looking for a cure for malaria. "He's a hero. He absolutely is," she says of him. We consider her a pleasure revolutionary for her joyful novels, and for being smart enough to get into med school, but daring enough to drop out to write romance novels.

AN INTERVIEW WITH JULIA QUINN:

How did it happen that you went to Harvard and then ended up writing romance novels?
JULIA: I took the SATs when I was thirteen as part of a study with Johns Hopkins. I got a 490 on the verbal, which I think is pretty typical if you're thirteen, but I got a 700 on the math, which was really striking. I was only the twentieth girl who had done this. And so I was actually identified very young as a math person. It's a big problem that it's not cool for girls to be good at math and science. I rebelled against that to a certain degree because I really liked other stuff, such as the school plays.

I went to a prestigious boarding school on a full scholarship, and I decided I wanted to go to Harvard. My father was the only person in his high school to go to a private college, actually, and the first person in town to go to Harvard. They threw him a parade. *[laughter]*

I did write a novel while I was in high school, a teen romance. I was reading these teen romances over the summer because it was just fun, I liked them. And my dad who is a bit of an intellectual, said, "Give me one good reason to read those."

So I said, "Well, I'm reading it for vocabulary words."

And he said, "OK, you find me one word in that book that you didn't already know."

And I couldn't do it, which is partly the books' fault and partly my fault because I had a pretty good vocabulary. And I said, "I'm doing research because I'm going to write one." And so he said, "OK," and he sat me down in front of his computer and I started writing. I wrote about half the book the first summer and half the book the next summer. I sent it to one place to try to get published. I wrote what I thought was a really interesting letter saying this book will feel so much more authentic because it's written by a teenager. I got a rejection back so quickly that I'm convinced they just looked at the letter and said, "She's sixteen. This can't be any good." And I was very discouraged.

But, when I was applying to Harvard and I was filling out my application there was a choice of listing the five most meaningful books you ever read, or discussing the most meaningful book. So I discussed the book I wrote. And I'm convinced to this day that that's how I got into Harvard. Because that was the only thing that made me different than anyone else. So I think romance writing actually got me into Harvard. *[laughter]*

Why did you decide to pursue medicine?
JULIA: I had a great time at Harvard and didn't really know what I wanted to do. At the end of my senior year I had been working as a peer counselor in a quasi-medical field, as a contraceptive counselor, and I had to take a science distribution requirement, evolutionary biology. I just love genetics and all that stuff, and I felt I had been rebelling against science for so long, maybe I would like to go into medicine. I wanted to feel like I knew what I wanted to do. So I spent the next couple years doing my science requirements. And the whole time I was doing this, I was writing a romance novel, because I really liked to read them. I don't know what got my butt in the chair the first time, but I enjoyed it and I liked it and I was working on it. I wanted to write the book and sell it and sold the book the same month I got into Yale medical school. And I ended up deferring medical school for two years.

I was twenty-six when I had what I call a mid-twenties crisis. I had just gotten married and all of a sudden, I was thinking, "Oh my gosh, if this writing thing doesn't work, I'm not qualified to do anything!" *[laughter]* And so I threw myself on the mercy of the Yale admissions board. I went for about two months, and then I realized that it wasn't the right thing. I hated the sense that you were never caught up. I'm always behind on my books, but once a year, I'm not behind and that's a really nice feeling. And with medicine you're *always* behind, you're never caught up on everything you need to do.

Do you feel that there is a stigma against romance?
JULIA: Yeah.

How do you feel about that? How do you deal with that?
JULIA: I haven't felt it as much as some of my colleagues. There are plenty of Harvard students reading romances under the covers. *[laughter]* But it is so far out of my friends' experience that it's intriguing to them. So I don't run into it that much, but I have had people say to me things like, "Wait a minute, so does somebody write your plots? Like, give you an outline and then you write it?" No, these are real books, I write, I do it all myself. Some people will say, "Well, don't you want to write a real book?" They are real books. *[laughter]* And one that I haven't heard directly but I've heard other people say is, "Oh, you're reading a romance because you need more romance in your life." Are you reading a mystery because you need more murder in your life? *[laughter]* And then a question I get a lot, which probably shouldn't bother me, but it does a little bit is: "Well, do you read romances?" To me I always interpret it a little bit as "Are you just doing this because you can? And you can make money?" And no, I actually do. I really like the genre. I like it and it's something that suits my particular writing talents.

Why do you think there is a stigma against romances?
JULIA: There are several reasons. The obvious one is the covers, which are changing but they were horrible. The awful clinches, anatomically incorrect, with the clothes coming off. And the irony of that is that they were originally designed to appeal to men: when romance really burst on to the scene, huge numbers of books would be sold through independent distributors who were racking the drugstores and the

bookstores, and they were all men. So you put a book cover on that's got this woman with huge boobs coming out of her dress, and the guys are like, "That's a good cover. We'll buy a hundred thousand of those." *[laughter]* Then it's a self-fulfilling prophesy because they buy a hundred thousand, it sells really well and then all the books now have these horrible covers. We're getting away from that and although as much as I hate the covers, I do have to say that when you're starting out they can be very helpful because they do immediately identify the book as a romance and they help the core readership find you.

Another reason there is a stigma is that they are by women for women. The irony is that a lot of things that are by women for women also get looked down upon by women. There is also a stigma because they deal with things on an emotional level and they have happy endings. People, I think, can be afraid of their emotions.

How would you describe your typical reader?

JULIA: They're really different. I think a better way, rather than say a typical one, may be to describe the most common type I see: a mom, she might work, she might stay at home, she's got some little kids, married. But I also get emails from highly educated women. Sometimes you notice they have an educational email address. I had somebody who's in the department of something at MIT. [It was] one of those moments where I was thinking to myself, I don't even know what that is. *[laughter]* Some of the nicest letters I've ever gotten are letters from women that say, "I never liked to read before I found romance novels because I couldn't find anything that was fun." I overheard a woman who said that she had been functionally illiterate until she discovered romance novels and it gave her a reason to really finally learn how to read. So, there's a huge spectrum. I value them all, really.

What are your personal pleasures?

JULIA: I love reading. Going to the spa. *[laughter]* I really do. Getting a massage, and my toes done, things like that. I love holding my child's hand. I love when a story comes on NPR that I love so much that I have to park in front of my house and listen to the rest of it. And then everybody stares at you funny. *[laughter]* I like going out to a really good restaurant. And I like to cook when I feel I have the time. I like to swim laps. I love the feeling of getting my desk cleared off. I don't much like clearing it off, but I like when it's cleared. I've paid all the bills.

I love when I'm driving by myself and a really good song comes on and I play it really loud and I sing along to it. Sometimes I'll be driving along, and I'll just be struck by this feeling, wow life is good, look what I have. In the end, I'm just very happy, I'm a happy person.

CHAPTER 27

Laugh a Lot

Pleasure has a sense of humor

WHY YOU NEED A SENSE OF HUMOR TO
SURVIVE IN THIS WORLD—MARIA

My brother David was hysterically funny. He didn't always intend to be funny, but it seemed he couldn't fight it—so he spent lots of time purposefully being funny. He'd write outrageously fictional letters. He'd tell stories that were delightfully mean. Sometimes we would just make funny noises and cry with happy tears. Like all really funny people, David was covering up a lot of hurt and pain, like the fact that he knew he wasn't living up to my father's ideal and didn't really want to.

Only after he died did I realize just how much his humor had carried our family through. Suddenly, there was no laughter. No jokes. No ridiculous stories. It wasn't just that we were sad and depressed. (We were, but he would have made jokes about that, too.) It was that David had been such a center of attention with his humor that the rest of us hadn't had to worry about making an effort.

The year after David died I hung out with my dad a little bit more than usual. Maya and I had moved to Washington, D.C., for my first real job and Dad would come down on business and stop by and take us out for dinner. I began to realize that I could make him laugh. That was a moment of enlightenment for me. His laughter was like a jolt of happy gas into my lungs. I felt powerful. I finally understood why my brother had enjoyed being so funny . . . it was the best way he could please my father. Plus, laughing just feels good.

When I met Lou, part of the reason I knew he was The One was that he got my sense of humor. We both worked in the circulation department at Rodale, and weren't dating yet. Our cubicles were right next to each other and throughout the day we would send comments through the wall and over it on little Post-it note basketballs. I don't remember exactly what it was he said or did, but something made me laugh, get up, and walk over to his cubicle to say to him, "You know, you are just as weird as I am." He did not deny it.

Lou is a tough one to get a laugh out of, though. He smiles a lot and laughs easily for his buddies. But I have to really work to get it out of him. And when I am finally rewarded by his uncontainable bark of laughter, it feels like I've won an Emmy for Best Comedy Writer for a Marriage.

Lou really helped me clean up my act. He doesn't like teasing, which can be hurtful and mean, and I don't either. So I've tried really hard to not be funny at others' expense or point out other people's flaws and laugh at them. That has taken a while and occasionally I have relapses. I think I watched too many *Three Stooges* episodes growing up, but the sight of any sort of slapstick physical stuff sends me into hysterics. Lou hasn't been able to cure me of that. My humor tends towards the dry side. Really dry. So dry, in fact, that Lou sometimes hasn't realized I was making a joke and has thought I'm being serious. For a few years I actually had to raise my hand every time I made a joke just so he knew I was making one.

Now we have settled into a comfortable life, finding humor where and whenever we can get it. Sometimes Eve and I watch the "Funniest Animal Videos" before bed. Or we just watch our dog, the new kitten, or the squirrels outside. That's usually good for a few laughs. Thursday night comedy TV is a sacred time—please don't call between the hours of eight and ten. When in doubt and slightly depressed we rent really stupid comedies like *Dude, Where's My Car?* or *Cheaper by the Dozen*. I *always* feel better after a movie like that. I know that if I'm laughing, I'm still alive.

LAUGH A LOT—MAYA

Once upon a time my friend caught this guy in the act of cheating on her. When she called me, I tried to be soothing and listened closely to see if I could detect tears. But after a minute or two I gave up because I was the one in tears—from laughing so much. "You are so funny" I said. "But how can you be making jokes at a time like this?"

"Humor heals the pain," she said.

And it does—at least, a certain kind of humor. Humor can be a weapon or an olive branch; you have to be very careful when wielding it. Over the years I have cultivated a sense of humor that ensures I am laughing a lot. I laugh when people bonk their heads or trip (as long as they don't get hurt. Pain is not funny to me). My favorite joke is "A guy walked into a bar . . . ouch!" Any sort of bathroom related joke or story makes me laugh. Sexual jokes and puns make me giggle. My friends say I have the mind and sense of humor of an adolescent boy, and frankly, I must agree. I love a good word pun, like "Liquor, I don't even know her!" On that note, take a look at my pride and joy, a list of "words that sound dirty but aren't."

When taking one of my first subway rides, I got on the train in the wrong direction, which was stopping at places I had never even heard of. I knew how scared I was when I couldn't even laugh at the "Rector Street" stop.

Once, my parents were discussing what kind of new car to get. My dad suggested a Volvo and they asked for my opinion. I said that every time I see a Volvo or hear the word Volvo, I think of *vulva* and it amuses me. We didn't get a Volvo, and in our house the make is now referred to as "those very box-shaped cars."

I once read that a certain Eastern sect considered laughter a form of enlightenment. For a moment, when you laugh, you just get IT. There is no thinking it through, just immediate comprehension and a spontaneous burst of laughter.

DO IT: HAVE A COMEDY WEEKEND AND SEE HOW IT FEELS

A comedy weekend should be funny, which may not be as easy as it sounds. Lots of people have different ideas of what is funny, so you have to find your own.

A good place to start is on the TV. Check out Comedy Central, cartoons, and old episodes of Seinfeld. Our personal favorites are old episodes of *The Young Ones*, *Pee Wee's Playhouse*, and *Three Stooges*.

Next, rent some movies. Most people don't find Woody Allen movies as funny as the purely goofy classics, like *Caddyshack* and *There's Something About Mary*. The essence of highbrow tends to be its lack of a sense of humor. So lower yourself, ladies. It's funny down there. If you don't laugh in *Cheaper by the Dozen* when the kid throws up and then slips and falls in it—you need a comedy intervention.

Read some funny stories, like anything by David Sedaris or Erma Bombeck.

Play some games. Kickball, charades, tag. Get yourself moving. That often makes it easier to laugh.

Read the comic strips. We find it funny that *The New York Times* has absolutely zero funnies and *The Washington Post* has three full pages. Would anyone read *The New Yorker* if it wasn't for the cartoons?

Check out your local comedy club. In Emmaus, Pennsylvania, the local sandwich deli shop turns into a comedy club at night. That, in itself, is sort of funny.

Last, but not least, go to your local supermarket or Hallmark store and read the goofy greeting cards. They aren't all funny, but usually you can get one or two good laughs. Buy the best ones and send them to people who are simply not expecting it. They just might get a good laugh, too.

LIST: WORDS THAT SOUND DIRTY THAT AREN'T

Dictum
Volvo
Kumquat
Asinine
Crotchety
Anything with *cock*: cocktail, coccyx, peacock
Angina
Rectify, rectory
Shiitake
Sirloin
Uranus

Pianist
Penal
Shih-Tzu
Tampa
Heinous
Pusillanimous
Bangkok
Masticate
Gaelic
Sacrament
Ramification
Hormone

IN HER OWN VOICE: LUCILLE BALL

"The Puritan idea that everything pleasurable is somehow bad almost ruined for me the first joys of our big *I Love Lucy* success. The hardest thing for me was getting used to the idea that I deserved it."

"Here is what I advise any young struggling actresses today: The important thing is to develop as a woman first, and a performer second. You wouldn't prostitute yourself to get a part, not if you're in your right mind. You won't be happy, whatever you do, unless you're comfortable with your own conscience. Keep your head up, keep your shoulders back, keep your self-respect, be nice, be smart. And remember that there are practically no "overnight" successes. Before that brilliant hit performance came ten, fifteen, sometimes twenty years in the salt mines, sweating it out."

"I have a theory about the assists we get in life. Only rarely can we repay those people who helped us, but we can pass that help along to others."

"I believe that we're as happy in life as we make up our minds to be."

"The *I Love Lucy* show was love personified. It was little domestic spats and upsets happily concluded, an exaggeration of American life that came out all right."

"Knowing what you can *not* do is more important than knowing what you *can* do. In fact, that's good taste."

"You really have to love yourself to get anything done in this world."

PLEASURE REVOLUTIONARY: LUCILLE BALL—SHE BROKE ALL THE RULES AND MADE 'EM LAUGH

Like all of our pleasure revolutionaries, Lucy wasn't perfect. She had an awful temper. Even though she had craved children desperately, she was obsessed with her work, and her kids felt mostly ignored and unloved. In her final years, she drank too much, and was crabby and depressed about aging.

But she made America laugh. Lucy was television's first wife and mother. Far from being a June Cleaver, *Leave It to Beaver* ideal, she was sassy, a troublemaker. Most importantly she was *ambitious*. She wasn't content to sit around and crochet. She wanted to do things. Each episode on the *I Love Lucy* show ended with her failing in her ambition and husband Ricky Ricardo forgiving her transgressions, but in real life Lucy accomplished her goals (and Desi didn't always forgive her).

Lucy had a tough childhood. Born in 1911 to a young mother who was happily married, Lucy's first four years were joyful. Then her father died, thrusting her pregnant mother into a life of poverty. In her memoir, found after she died, she wrote: "I'm known among comediennes as a stunt girl who will do anything. . . . Perhaps my willingness to be knocked off a twenty-foot pedestal or shot down a steamship funnel goes back to my earliest, happiest days with my father. I *knew* he was going to catch me; I *wasn't* going to get hurt."

Her mother, depressed and in need of a job, left her baby son with her own parents and sent Lucy to live with her paternal grandparents, devout Christians, whose home was severe and loveless. "Anything that gave pleasure lapsed into one of the seven deadly sins and was therefore 'devil's bait,'" she said. "Nothing in this life was ever to be enjoyed, only endured." She credits those hard times with teaching her how to live in a world of imagination, which she believes was critical for her becoming an actress.

Eventually Lucy returned to live with her mother, brother, and maternal grandparents. But then a weird tragic confluence of events happened. Her beloved grandmother died. Her grandfather bought her brother a gun. While they were practicing in the yard, a little girl neighbor asked to try it and accidentally shot another neighbor boy in the back. The little boy was paralyzed from the waist down. The family sued, and after a long hard trial, Lucy's grandfather lost everything—including the house they lived in.

Lucy buried herself in acting in high school, moved to New York City afterwards to go to acting school, but got kicked out after the first semester because she couldn't dance or sing. At one point she only had four pennies to her name. Then she started getting modeling jobs (she even did a topless modeling job), but came down with a strange undiagnosed leg problem where she couldn't walk and had to go home for a year to recover.

But she went back. She got other modeling jobs—including one for an illustration for Chesterfield cigarettes, which led to her first big break in Hollywood. After a few years struggling in Hollywood, Ginger Rogers's mother took her under her wing and made her straighten her teeth and dye her hair a different color. Gradually, slowly, Lucy became the queen of B movies. She got involved in radio at twenty-eight, making $1,000 a week and looking for love.

About this time she met Desi Arnaz, a Cuban playboy who had been raised on plantations, boats, and horses by two loving, wealthy parents. After the revolution in Cuba, however, they had to leave everything behind. It wasn't love at first sight, Lucy later said. "It took five minutes."

Their relationship was stormy, and friends gave it less than a year, but they married and, in spite of lots of fights, stayed married for twenty years. After ten years, they had children. All the while they were both working like mad, trying to find a way to work together, and Lucy even was hospitalized for exhaustion a few times.

In 1951, Desi and Lucy were offered a chance to do a TV series based on a radio show that Lucy had worked on about a married couple. Because she was pregnant with her first child, they didn't want to move to New York to do a live show, so they created their own studio in Hollywood, named Desilu. In collaboration, they hired writers, and Desi directed and managed the studio. The result, I Love Lucy, became the number one show in America. On Monday nights stores closed, telephones stopped ringing, and taxis disappeared from the streets. Two years later when Lucy got pregnant again, she became the first woman to be pregnant on TV or the stage. When little Ricky was born, more than a million people sent cards, flowers, and good wishes. They won Emmys. They got an $8 million deal from Philip Morris.

As the show wound down, their studio business got huge. But Desi started drinking a lot and their fighting was destroying their marriage. Lucy and Desi finally got divorced. Both married other, less volatile people soon after, but they stayed in touch and shared custody of the kids. When Desi decided to retire as studio head, Lucy took the job and became the first woman to run a Hollywood studio.

The romantic in us likes to believe that they were meant to be together . . .

The last time Lucy went to see Desi, when he was dying of lung cancer, they laughed and talked just like old times. When she got up to go he asked her where she was going.

"Home," she said.

"You *are* home," he said.

And when Lucy died a few months later, her husband said: "I guess she's happy now. She's with Desi."

CHAPTER 28

Believe In the Power of Love

*Pleasure has provided you
with the only tool you will ever need
to protect you on your journey*

TRUE LOVE—MARIA

In the beginning of my spiritual journey I was convinced that I could find a common thread running through all the major religions and I suspected that maybe it would be love. Yet I was shocked to find that each religion, in its own way, is rife with inconsistencies, violence, and political ambitions. Love was not the common thread but the desire to control people seemed to be. Nonetheless, I was determined to get at the root of what drives us all.

When I was little, in the late 1960s, I remember my family being called "radicals."

"What's a radical?" I asked my Dad.

"Let's go look it up," he said. I will never forget the understanding and pride I had when I looked at that definition. According to *Webster's*, a radical was a root part, a basic principle, relating to the origin of something. I remember that definition every time I am faced with a dilemma. I ask myself— what's the root and the origin of it all? So many

you want to worship, you have to play it really loud and dance around in your underwear and love every joyous minute of it. If you are a member, you know the joy of a chorus that is really a chorus, your loud and off-key voice included, you appreciate the sacred key change at the bridge, you know your heart beats in four quarter time, you know that love songs never grow old.

I was born in the same year as MTV. We grew up together. Maybe I did watch *Sesame Street*, but I remember music videos far more vividly. I was obsessed. When I was three, I insisted everyone call me Michael, as in Jackson. Apparently, I did a freakishly good Paula Abdul dance routine. I knew every Madonna lyric and video. I thought Jon Bon Jovi was a God (I mean really, how could you not?).

I distinctly remember one day—I must have been six or seven—asking my mom why every song I heard was about LOVE—requited, unrequited, broken hearts, happy hearts, longing, lust, infatuation, satisfaction—love. "Because that's the one thing everyone can relate to," she said. Truer words were never spoken. That is the day of my baptism, the day I was born again, the day I accepted love and pop music into my heart.

Fast forward a few years to the time one of my best friends and I were on the long drive to Chicago. I was doing the driving, and I told her to be the DJ and put on some upbeat music to keep me going. "I think you'll love this," she said, putting some music on. And then she fell asleep while I listened to a lone drunk man sing about broken hearts, being poor, hung over, and suffering, while he played what sounded like a two string untuned guitar and tapping his foot out of time. This was most certainly not what I had in mind. But she had fallen asleep with the CD player in her lap and I couldn't change the music.

As I listened to the old man wail, I thought about what my friend and I had been talking about during those long driving hours—her love life, or lack of it. An interesting contradiction; she wanted to fall in love, to have a boyfriend, and yet she routinely disses pop music, romance novels, and romantic comedies—basically everything that celebrates the stomach-flipping, heart-pounding, shouting out one's joy from the rooftops aspect of love.

All songs are love songs—from the united chorus of a pop song to the solitary wailing of the blues. But there is something truly mys-

DO IT: SPREAD THE SEEDS OF LOVE

This one feels surprisingly good.

1.   Smile at strangers on the street and in other cars.

2.   Give someone a gift even though it's not a special occasion.

3.   Sign your notes, letters, and emails with love, xxoo.

4.   Be nice to strangers when in stressful situations—long lines, traffic jams.

5.   Tell everyone you love that you love them . . . and give them a hug.

If you were on a plane and it was going to crash and you had a cell phone and you could call anyone and say anything, what would it be? Most likely it would not be, "Honey, don't forget to take out the trash." Most likely you would want to tell people that you love them. Why wait?

LIST: SOUNDTRACK TO THE PLEASURE REVOLUTION

Selection One: *FIND YOURSELF*

I Have Confidence—*Sound of Music* soundtrack

This One's for the Girls—Martina McBride

Extraordinary—Liz Phair

This Woman's Work—Kate Bush

When I Was a Boy—Dar Williams

The Pleasure Is All Mine—Bjork

Hey Ya—OutKast

Express Yourself—Madonna

Hallelujah—Jeff Buckley

The Good Stuff—Kenny Chesney

tical and powerful about a love song you can sing along to, that
know instinctively even though you may be hearing it for the
time. That's what a good pop song is. You can dismiss it as formu
or you can recognize the power of an instant connection. It is
that a mother bonds with her newborn in the first three minutes
it any coincidence that most pop songs are three minutes lon
don't think so.

Pop songs on the radio and TV are good but there is nothing l
live concert. Nothing. There is nothing more profound, humbling
exalting than a stadium full of *thousands* of people experiencing
singing along to the same song. Buy U2's *Rattle and Hum* album
play the live version of "Pride" and listen to thousands of p
singing the line "IN THE NAME OF LOVE" at the top of their l
singing the *oh-oh-oh-uh* with Bono and perfect strangers. It is co
trated passion, love, release, joy, and hope. Even though there ar
of painful and rotten things in the world and there is oppressio
segregation and differences in sex, sexual orientation, race, natio
violence, class, education, and politics, if thousands of people ca
the same love song together all is not lost. As long as we have
happy pop songs, there is hope.

The girls in the front row weep and sob and scream and pul
hair in a state of pure ecstasy, like when statues of the Virgin
weep, or a pious, devoted Catholic manifests stigmata on his han
a blessed and holy miracle. I didn't think I could ever really let
that at a concert but I deeply admired and envied people wh
Then, one night, it happened to me.

The lights went down, the audience roared, and the openin
of *Vogue* blared out of the speakers. All of a sudden, I was eigh
old again, reliving the moment of excitement and anticipatio
my mom let me stay up past my bedtime to watch the world d
the *Vogue* video. And the stage lights came on, the musi
through, and Madonna stepped on stage. Oh My God. Bef
even hit the chorus, the tears were skipping down my face. I
that girl in the music video. Those tears were the renewal of n
and the reaffirmation of my faith in the joy and power of p
love.

Selection Two: *CREATE THE WORLD AROUND YOU*

What It Feels Like for a Girl—Madonna

She Will Be Loved—Maroon 5

When You Come—Crowded House

I Don't Know How to Love Him—*Jesus Christ Superstar* soundtrack

I Believe in a Thing Called Love—The Darkness

I Will Survive—Gloria Gaynor

You Gotta Be—Des'ree

Wild Horses—Charlotte Martin

Love Is Everything—Jane Siberry

I'm Like a Bird—Nelly Furtado

I Believe in Love—Dixie Chicks

Selection Three: *LIVE THE LIFE YOU HAVE ALWAYS DESIRED*

Think Pink—Kay Thompson

La La Love You—Pixies

Like a Prayer—Madonna

Think Pink—*Funny Face* soundtrack

Sowing the Seeds of Love—Tears for Fears

The Heart Asks Pleasure First—*The Piano* soundtrack

Prelude, Op..28, No.4 in E Minor—Chopin

When I Grow Up —Michele Shocked

Days Go By—Keith Urban

(What's So Funny 'bout) Peace, Love, and Understanding—Elvis Costello

IN HER OWN VOICE: CAROL GILLIGAN

"Pleasure is a sensation written into our bodies, the emotion of delight and joy."

"I came to see love as a courageous act and pleasure as its harbinger."

"Patriarchy drains pleasure because hierarchy leads us to cover vulnerability."

"It's not possible to talk about trauma without talking about pleasure, the way life returns even in the face of the most terrible adversity, like a plant pushing its way through the sidewalk."

PLEASURE REVOLUTIONARY: CAROL GILLIGAN— *THE BIRTH OF PLEASURE*

We discovered Carol Gilligan while we were writing our book proposal. Our agent asked us to put together a competitive analysis and she said: "How is your book going to be different from *The Birth of Pleasure*?" Huh? We had never heard of it. So, off to the Amazon we went. A few days later we were stunned by its powerful message and its validation of our ideas about the importance of pleasure, and the power of stories to define our existence. Once again, the universe seemed to guide us right to where we needed to be.

Carol Gilligan is currently a professor at New York University, having been a professor at Harvard for thirty-four years, and its first gender studies professor. With a Ph.D. in psychology from Harvard, in the early 1980s she wrote the groundbreaking book *In a Different Voice: Psychological Theory and Women's Development*, which explored the unique power and difference of women's ways of expressing themselves, which had not previously been explored in scientific and academic studies.

The Birth of Pleasure reveals the stories that our culture relies on to control our lives and expectations. For instance, one story our culture tells is that love is tragic. "The tragic story where love leads to loss and pleasure is associated with death was repeated over and over again in operas, folk songs, the blues, and novels. We [all cultures] were in love with a tragic story of love. It was 'our story.'"

Why is that? It's because love threatens the control and power of patriarchy. "The sacrifice of love is a common feature of patriarchal religions and cultures," she writes. "We learn it, repeat it symbolically in the stories of Abraham and Isaac, Jephthe and his daughter, Agamemnon and Iphigenia, as well as the Oedipus tragedy. A parent willing to sacrifice a child is a demonstration of loyalty to God." When women are seen as property and children as a means of transferring wealth and a father's lineage, love is a terrible threat. Love means people might marry people of differing classes, religions, castes or nations. Love means girls and boys have a will and mind of their own and may do something different from their parents' wishes. (Think Romeo and Juliet.) The tragic love story is the perfect way of scaring people into obedience. It's the Pandora's box that must not be opened . . . or else . . . the world will end! Because, yes, for the patriarchs, it *will* end.

It's why, in so many cultures, adultery (for *women* only) is a punishable crime. Gilligan recounts that in the early days of patriarchy the Roman emperor Augustus passed a law making adultery a crime and sending all adulteresses (except the prostitutes) to an island. For one of the first times in recorded Western history, the wives revolted, and all registered themselves as prostitutes! But in other cultures at the time—including the Jewish culture—adulteresses were legally stoned to death. The Old Testament sanctions it.

The title of Gilligan's book, *The Birth of Pleasure*, refers to the story of Psyche and Eros. Throughout human history, stories have celebrated the power of love. Often they showed that disobedience of cultural "rules" is the secret to finding love. Venus, the goddess of love, decides that a mortal girl named Psyche, who rivals her in beauty, must be made to suffer. She bids her son, Eros, the god of love, to shoot off his arrow in the most wretched man so that Psyche will fall in love with someone horrible. Instead, after one look at her, Eros shoots himself in the heart. Because he doesn't want to get in trouble with his mother, Eros forbids Psyche to see who he really is and they marry in complete darkness. Each night he comes to her and they make passionate, erotic love. Psyche gets pregnant, and her jealous sisters tell her she has to find out who the father really is, because he could be a monster and she might give birth to a little monster.

So one night Psyche lights the lamp as Eros sleeps to see who her husband really is. Stunned by his beauty, she falls even more deeply in love, but she accidentally awakens him and he leaves—angry that she didn't trust him and that his dangerous secret has been revealed. Psyche follows him all over the world and into the underworld before he finally gives in to his own love for her. Before Venus will let them live happily ever after, however, she gives Psyche a series of impossible tasks to perform. Each time, nature comes to her aid. She accomplishes her final task, but then falls into a deep sleep because she accidentally opens Persephone's "day's worth of beauty in a jar" (not kidding!). This time, Eros comes to her rescue. They get married again. This time Psyche is given immortal life and Venus dances at the wedding.

Eros and Psyche give birth to a daughter. And her name is Pleasure.

Gilligan writes that "Jungian analysts have seen the Psyche myth as an archetype, a reflection in the collective unconscious of the soul's affinity for love. I saw it more specifically as capturing a possibility that arises when a moment of resistance in girls' development converges with a moment of liberation in cultural history and reveals the potential for love to dissolve social hierarchy and give birth to pleasure."

If *The Birth of Pleasure* were just about stories, it would still be a perfect book for us. But what makes it pack a wallop is that Gilligan has also spent her life as a psychologist studying how and when girls and boys lose their natural voices, submerging them and sacrificing them to the god of patriarchy.

When we are babies, we know instinctively that love is the good stuff. It's what makes us healthy and happy and safe. It's what makes us strong. But the culture roots out of us the feeling of safe love. In her previous studies on girls, Gilligan found that "One confiding relationship, meaning a relationship where one is invited to speak one's heart and mind freely, offers the best protection against most forms of psychological trouble, especially in times of stress." When she started to study boys, she found that around the age of five, parents start to feel concern that a boy's sensitivity will lead to trouble on the playground so they start to toughen him up. In some cultures, this is the age when boys are separated from their mothers, and when boys (and parents and teachers) start playing "good guy" vs. "bad guy." The good boys fit in, don't get into trouble. The bad boys can't be controlled and don't follow the rules. The close, loving relationship gets cut off. "The sacrifice of relationship [with the parents] is the ritual of initiation into patriarchy," she states. But more and more, parents are unwilling to make that sacrifice. "In their own ways, with greater or lesser degrees of conviction and fear, these parents of sons are coming to the discovery that love erodes patriarchy."

For girls, the loss of relationship and voice happens later—in adolescence. Girls are allowed to be strong and confident until age eleven or twelve. Then the culture tells them it's time to get real, to give up their girlish fantasies and dreams. Often, this causes a dissociation—a split between their inner being that still wants to believe and their outer being that wants to fit in and be a part of the group. This is the time when cruel playground games make a girl choose whether she wants to join the world order or stay apart. It's when her face (like boys at a younger age) turns expressionless and masks her true feelings. It's when she starts speaking in questions instead of statements. The experience of loss is so deep that it often leads to depression, eating disorders, and "acting out."

How do we get out of it? "In dissociation, we literally don't know what we know; and the process of recovery, now illuminated by the biological and psychological studies of trauma, centers on the recovery of voice and, with it, the ability to tell one's story." So basically, if you want to reconnect and reassociate with your true self, if you want to live a life of pleasure and love, you have to write and rewrite the story of your life. We have to open up our hearts to the power of love.

Gilligan writes: "The mystery of love will never be unraveled. . . . But by uncovering truths about love in an ancient story, by exposing a long-standing social and literary history that leaves a knot in the psyche and exploring this knotted place in our souls, I found a path leading to pleasure and discovered it is also a road to freedom."

What's most fascinating to us, however, is the dissociation that Gilligan herself reveals that reflects the academic and intellectual divide that has yet to be crossed. When she says "Collectively, we have moved to an edge of possibility; it has become possible to envision a democracy that is not patriarchal; *it is more difficult to imagine a love that is passionate without becoming tragic*" (italics added). HELLO! Romance novels! Never once in Gilligan's book does she refer to the vast underground of romance readers and writers. It's like the flame that refuses to die, even if it must be lit in secret. Nora Roberts has probably sold more books than Shakespeare, but does she get a high school or college class devoted to her? No. We find it shocking that Gilligan could write a whole book on the role of stories in our life and not mention the single largest selling segment of publishing that actually supports her claims.

Often during that terrible teen initiation period, when girls first turn to reading romances, it's accompanied by a sense of shame and illicit pleasure. *Romances are the illegitimate child of our patriarchal society.* They are the "love child." I think it's a positive thing that there is no shame these days in having a child out of wedlock. When I made the announcement I was having Maya out of wedlock, shame burned in my face. I felt that the best option would have been to disappear to some remote European village where I could have passed myself off as a widow. Today, while teen pregnancy is a "problem," it's out in the open.

All these things are connected. It's time to legitimize love. Legitimize romance. Legitimize romance novels. Legitimize women and children without fathers. It's time to free our sons and daughters from the vicious cycle of initiation that leads to the loss of their joy and their voices. It's time to give birth to pleasure.

The Birth of Pleasure is a great book. And Carol Gilligan is a true pleasure revolutionary. Now, if she would just read a few romances . . .

CHAPTER 29

Live Each Age to Its Fullest
Pleasure knows no age

**BARE YOUR BELLY AT TWENTY, WEAR BIG
JEWELRY AFTER FORTY—MARIA**

Like most women, I've had mixed feelings about aging. Although mine were sort of backwards. When I was younger I distinctly remember wanting to be an old lady. Old ladies seemed so damn sassy and free and they wore outrageous jewelry and seemed so interesting. I would look at my smooth white hands and wish they were gnarly and wrinkled like my grandmothers' or like old Navajo women who'd spent their whole lives in the desert sun. My grandmother always used to say I was born old.

But now that my hands are starting to gnarl and my boobs are starting to sink I can't help but say to myself, "What the hell was I thinking?" I wonder if I appreciated my younger days and my younger body enough. I wonder if I am ready to age.

I used to swear to myself that I would not be one of "those" women who fight aging tooth and nail. You know the ones: they wear miniskirts in their seventies. They become obsessed with plastic surgery and hair dye. They refuse to tell their age or, even worse, they complain and cry that they are not ready to become "grandmothers."

It's as if their aging process embarrasses them, and in trying to hide it, becomes even more embarrassing. Because I fear becoming one of those women, I've stubbornly refused to dye my hair, or consider plastic surgery even though my double chin is visible on TV.

One of the first articles I ever wrote was an interview with a Scottish doctor who had done research on eccentricity that has stayed with me forever: Eccentrics live longer than regular folks. Men become eccentrics early on, but women tend to wait till the kids are grown to let their eccentricity manifest itself. It's as if they hold it in and stuff it down until it's safe to break free. I determined in that moment that I wasn't going to wait. And I'm so glad I didn't.

Looking back at my life, that positive knowledge about eccentrics helped free me to create a life I had dreamed about. It helped me to stay my true self through all the ups and downs. It made me less embarrassed to wear strange things or say what was really on my mind. It helped me to trust my inner voice, my instincts, and my heart.

I hope I'm lucky enough to become a real old lady. I'm going to make my homemade chicken soup for my grandkids (if I'm lucky enough to have any). We'll work in the garden together and I'll tell them stories of the olden days. I'll let them read age-inappropriate books they find in my library and get really really messy and dirty and not care. Then I'll let them all take baths together in the big Japanese tub and let them all fall asleep in my big fluffy bed.

But for now, I'm in my forties. I've started experimenting with wearing big jewelry (finally!). I care less and less what people think of me—although I still care. My hair is 30 percent gray. My chin is still double. But I've done what I have wanted to do and continue to, regardless of what the world thinks I should be doing. I'm defining my life in a way I want to.

Meanwhile I feel incredible gratitude that I've made it this far. I feel so thankful for every gift and every burden. Maybe because I've experienced the deaths of people close to me I realize just how precious each day is. As country music star Tim McGraw sings, I try to "Live like I was dying." I know that each seemingly unimportant conversation with any person could be my—or their—last. And I know I want it all to end well. It's so much easier to accept someone's death when you know she knew you loved her. And when your last moment together was one of kindness.

I'm sad that my kids will never know my dad as an old grandfather, or my brother as the eccentric old uncle. So I owe it to them and to me to take what I learned from their lives and deaths and apply it—live each age, each day to its fullest.

THE JOY OF BEING TWENTY—MAYA

*J*oy in the city comes from the little things: picnics in a park, staying out all night because you can, twenty-four-hour delis on every corner, Saturday brunch with the girls, walking past street corners where your favorite movie was filmed, museums, anything for sale, anything delivered at any hour, rock shows where you probably know someone in the band, cab rides late at night through the canyons of skyscrapers . . . Or maybe it comes from the big things: Having your whole life ahead of you, a place that offers every opportunity. New York is not the only city in the world to offer these things and lure young people away from small towns. Perhaps a city is alluring because there is something for everyone.

No matter where you are, being in your twenties is exciting. Generally, we live without family, spouse, children, or house. We have only ourselves and our dreams, combined with a freedom that still tastes new and fresh. And though it's different for everyone, some things are the same.

There is a tendency to think that twenty-something life in New York City is like a cheaper version of *Sex and the City*—smaller apartments, sans Manolos, and hipster hangouts. But one of my friends who grew up in the city has found her satisfaction in letting go of "notions of what it means to be living in New York in my twenties." She thought her life would be full of pricey cocktails and Soho lounges, and then realized she would much rather stay at home and rent a movie with her mom or do cartwheels in Central Park or flirt with the guy who works in the corner deli. She started listening to her mind and body instead of society. It's a hard shift to make. I myself had to finally admit that I had just as much fun, if not more, drinking cheap beers at a dive bar than standing in line behind the velvet rope at "cooler" places. Sometimes, the fun is just staying in one's tiny twenty-something apartment, thinking that if I pay this much in rent, I'm gonna stay in and get my money's worth.

Whether you live in a major city or a small town, in your twenties you are free to figure out how you really want to live your life. Another friend of mine likes being able to take risks that she might not be able to do at any other age. Most of us don't have any dependents, so this is the "decade during which you can still kind of screw up and it's still cute." We're young and employed (mostly) and can take risks with the money we earn, as we learn to pay taxes and rent and to budget so that we don't spend all our money on shoes.

Your options are always open and you really don't have to choose, and if you do, you can change your mind tomorrow night. Pretty much all of my friends agree that we'd better have it together once we hit thirty. Being in our twenties is a heady mixture of freedom and responsibility. We're bound to "nothing and no one" except ourselves and the opportunities to create the lives we want to be living.

DO IT: DEFINE YOUR DECADES AND DECIDE WHAT YOU WANT TO BE IN EACH ONE

Sit down with a tablet and write down an objective for each decade of your life. Map out where you want to be and what you want to be doing during each one. When do you want to have kids? When do you want to do all those things on all those lists you've made? When do you want to knuckle down and get serious about your health? When do you want to retire?

If you map it out and make it happen, you are the writer of the story of your life. Surprises will happen, but that will just add to the interest.

Ask yourself this: What will it take for you to get the most out of each age you live? What will you regret at fifty that you didn't do by thirty? And if you didn't make it to ninety or one hundred (or even if you did), what would make your life worth living?

LIST: HOW TO BE A HOYDEN

Early on in our romance reading days, we kept coming across the word *hoyden*. It was always used to describe the heroine in a part affectionate, part exasperated way. So one day we were looking it up in a book my

CHAPTER 30

Believe in Happy Endings
Pleasure is a path of optimism and hope

Cynicism is irresponsible.
—BARBARA KINGSOLVER

ALL THE LITTLE HAPPY ENDINGS—MARIA

One day Maya called me on her cell phone.

"You wouldn't believe the book I found. I am at the library—which you know I never go to—and I decided just to walk down this aisle and this old book caught my eye. Listen to this." And she read me an incredible paragraph that fit perfectly into our book.

"That is perfect!" I exclaimed.

"Maybe I'll never return it," she said.

"No. Who is the author and I'll buy it on Amazon."

"Helen Papashvily."

My heart skipped a beat.

"You are kidding," I said. It turns out the book that Maya accidentally found in the enormous NYU library—which was the perfect missing piece to our book—was written by one of my grandmother's best friends. Helen's husband George was a sculptor and my grandmother owned a few of his pieces.

I had a sudden vision of all of them, bohemian intellectuals in their grandfather created and edited called *The Synonym Finder.* It gave us such a great laugh we knew we had to share it with you:

Hoyden, *n.* 1. tomboy, romp, rowdy, termagant, roughneck, tough, whippersnapper, wench, hussy.—*adj.* 2. tomboyish, boyish, rough and tumble, rompish; boisterous, rambunctious, rowdy, unruly, wild; mischievous, troublesome, ill-behaved, hoydenish; unladylike, ill-bred, ill-mannered, ungenteel, rude; impudent, pert, saucy, fresh, cheeky, smart-alec, smart-alecky, minxish.

Basically, a hoyden is everything girls are told not to be . . . and everything a good man loves.

IN HER OWN VOICE: BEATRICE WOOD

"It is curious, but if one smiles, darkness fades."

"Celibacy is exhausting."

"Everybody wants freedom. We resent rules imposed from the outside, which can create chaos for the individual. But self-discipline is vital. We get no where without it."

"We develop through experience. Therefore, hardships and misfortunes challenge us. It is in overcoming mistakes that we touch the song of life."

"Perfection bores me."

"We are here on account of sex, though we do not understand its force. There is glory when the sexual force is used creatively, when it is open to the magic of the universe."

PLEASURE REVOLUTIONARY: BEATRICE WOOD— 105 YEARS OF CREATIVE PASSION

Here is a secret we only just discovered: The character of Rose in *Ti tanic* (the highest grossing movie of all time) was based on a re beefy but glamorous country outfits, sitting in the garden—the scent of chicken cooking in the kitchen and the cats (all twenty-nine of them) swirling about their ankles. And it all came full circle. As Steve Murphy says: "There are no coincidences." And as I always say: "Everything is connected."

This seemed just one of the many signposts from the universe that Helen and Nana wanted us to keep going—leading us towards a pleasure revolution. Real life is so much stranger and more interesting than fiction. This discovery was a little happy ending to our journey. Life is constantly moving—so there may never be the one grand happy ending. That's fine with me. I just want the little ones that happen all the time. The sun coming out after a storm. Falling into bed after a long hard good day (a cool summer breeze and the sound of crickets coming from the window), my children safe and snug in their beds. A wedding, a healthy birth, a surprise letter or package in the mail. Having delicious orgasmic sex on a Sunday afternoon. Coming home from a great vacation with a suitcase full of souvenirs. The sweet, tight goodnight hug from my little girl. A long, leisurely, peaceful family dinner. Finding the perfect book at the perfect moment . . . and then reading it in bed.

Life is so filled with magic and beauty. Once I surrendered to it and let go—followed the clues and signs—everything came together for me. I think back to the first time I found that prayer to Mary, and all the abandoned Marys who appeared before me wanting to be rescued. She's the one who got me started on all this. I might have rescued a few of her. But she rescued me, too.

I don't think of Mary as a Christian saint, or as Astarte, the villainess of the Old Testament. I think of her as just one of a long line of ancestresses leading all the way back to our genetic first mother, the black African woman whose DNA is still ours. The Goddess, Mary, the Black Virgin, Inanna, my Nana, and Helen Papashvily—they are all just saying the same thing. It is time.

It is time for women to remember who we really are. It is time for women to reclaim our power and our pleasure. It is time for women to save the world through the strength of our love. It's time for women to take back our long and illustrious heritage, without which the world would not exist. It is time for women to turn this tragic story into one with a happy ending . . . lots of little ones. It's time for a pleasure revolution.

It is time.

And it's my pleasure.

ALL THE HAPPY ENDINGS—MAYA

On my absolute final bit of research for my absolute final assignment of college, I went on my third trip in four years to the library to check out a book. Actually it was the first visit to borrow a book, since I'd been there before only to use the bathroom or meet a friend. Being so inexperienced, I forgot the reference number, and wasn't about to try to figure out how to look it up, so I decided to wander around until I found the book I needed. This was kind of ridiculous, since the NYU library is eight stories high and occupies most of a city block. I justified this by thinking "there must be a reason for this. I bet I'm supposed to just stumble on a book I never knew I needed." Maybe because I started looking for that book, I found it.

It's called *All the Happy Endings*. This was my IT book. On my daily phone call with my mum, I told her about it, and we decided the universe was trying to tell me something. I must admit, I didn't read the whole thing, since I didn't have the time, but I skipped to the last paragraph, and lordy am I glad I did. And this is what it said:

> For slowly and inefficiently the old social patterns do dissolve and resolve into new ones and a different and better kind of sex relationship begins to appear—the possibility of a true partnership that makes the fullest use of each individual and his particular gifts to complement and sustain and fulfill and advance the entity. Then when at last whole men and whole women are free to love as equals, they will find the real happy ending.

That is what we should all be aiming for. It starts with you, and your own personal pleasure, and it's not over until lives of pleasure are no longer revolutionary.

After I finish reading a romance novel, I feel happy and hopeful, and kind of sad that it's over at the same time. I crave more. And think of the millions of women who have read the same happy ending, and have probably felt the same way when they finished. One person's happy ending, either fictional or real, is everyone's happy ending.

Just for a minute imagine whole men and whole women loving each other as equals, with compassion and empathy and true understanding. They'll add up. They'll add up so much that all of a sudden a happy ending has become a happy beginning of a happy life and a happy world.

DO IT: CREATE YOUR OWN HAPPY ENDING. WHAT WOULD IT LOOK LIKE?

Is it true love or riches or both? Is it lots of children or complete freedom? Is it true love or true independence?

Sit or lie quietly in a place that you love and feel comfortable in. Close your eyes. Breathe deeply. Relax. Visualize yourself at the end of a long, happy, fruitful life. What does your life look like? Who is there with you? Where are you? What have you accomplished? What legacy are you leaving the world and your family?

Now, wake up. Take more deep breaths.

It's in your hands.

Make it happen.

LIST: THE INGREDIENTS FOR A HAPPY ENDING

The resolution of conflict. Life itself often provides the challenges and conflicts, but it's up to us to turn the struggle into an experience that makes us stronger and wiser.

Hope and faith. These beliefs often guide and comfort us through tough times. Keeping them close to the heart ensures that rough patches will be a phase, not an eternity.

No regrets. "What if's?" and "If only's" can sour even the happiest moment. When making a huge life decision, try to think how you'll feel about your choice years later. If you look back at something and cringe, let it go. There's nothing you can do about it, and that's OK.

Love. Ideally, your love will be returned and passionate. But if you just end up with a new love and respect for yourself alone, then that's a happy ending, too.

Satisfaction. Leave it to the boys to sing, "I can't get no satisfaction." Be the heroine to get her own satisfaction, sexual and otherwise.

New life. It could be the birth of a child, or the birth of a new woman—you. Each ending holds the seed of a new beginning.

IN HER OWN VOICE: THE REAL MARIA VON TRAPP

"But there is that certain something about wanting to do the will of God. If one is sincere and if one really wants to know what His will is, all one has to do is be quiet. Shut off television and radio, and in that silence one will always hear that still small voice in one's heart telling him what to do."

"Singing is like praying twice."

"There are times when it comes in handy when I can inform everybody that even a late vocation, like mine, will give the utmost joy and pleasure."

PLEASURE REVOLUTIONARY: MARIA VON TRAPP— CLIMBED EVERY MOUNTAIN, WHILE SINGING

Maria Von Trapp's story is the subject of the greatest feel-good movie of all time, *The Sound of Music*. You have heard all the songs—and probably even sung them. Even our agent, a New York intellectual, sneaks off once a year to watch it with her best friend. (She hasn't even told her husband about her secret habit.)

But what's the real story? What was the "real Maria" like? By all accounts, Maria Von Trapp's life could easily have read as a tragedy. She was a penniless orphan, abused by an insane stepfather. She was "forced" into marriage by her abbey. She and her seven stepchildren, two biological children (with one more on the way), and her husband escaped Nazi Austria leaving everything behind (home, possessions, money, toys). The very next day the borders were closed. They came to America with four dollars and had to make money to survive by singing. In her own words "Among the eight children God sent me, only three remained alive," although it's not clear whether the others were stillborn or miscarried. Her husband died of asbestos-related lung cancer when she was forty-two. She herself had a brain tumor, an almost fatal kidney infection, broke her back in a skiing fall, and broke all her ribs falling from a horse. Two of her stepchildren died before her. She sold all the rights to her story (with no royalties) for a few thousand dollars of immediate cash in 1947—so her family never saw more than that from what was arguably the most popular movie, play, and soundtrack of all time. A German company bought those rights, so somewhere in Germany someone has made hundreds of millions of dollars from it. Maria had to start a singing camp and hotel just to make money to keep her family going. She lost everything *again* when the hotel burned completely to the ground in 1980 (she escaped down a ladder in her pajamas into the frigid December night).

By her own account, she was a difficult wife. "I have a terrible temper, and I had thrown things across the room, yelled at the top of my voice, banged a door and, in order to make sure he understood what I meant, had opened the door again and slammed it again." She also indicates that she was a difficult mother, both domineering and distracted. And yet she was very happily married. She fell in love with the children first and they managed a proposal from their father. In a BBC documentary called *The Real Maria* she tells the funny story about how he asked her. Not knowing how to respond without hurting him she told him to wait a minute. She then ran into town and up to the abbey and asked the Reverend Mother what she should do. The Reverend Mother left the room and came back a few minutes later saying that she had prayed to the Holy Spirit and "found out it is the will of God that you marry the baron." Devastated by this order, she "sneaked" back to the villa. The baron, who was waiting in the front hall, asked, "And?"

She started sobbing and cried, "They have told me I have to marry you!" And so she did. Walking down the aisle, she was actually "blazing mad" that she had to go through with it. But a month later at Christmas Eve mass she let God and her husband back into her heart. She tried to act like his first wife, but he asked her to "please be yourself."

"From that moment on I was really in love," she said. "The real me—Maria—with my Georg."

The decision to leave Austria was difficult, but they decided it was better to lose all their possessions rather than lose their soul by staying under Hitler's rule.

Maria's determination led the family to become the most popular singing group of their time. After Georg died, it was also her resolve that led them to open a lodge, a singing camp, and a gift shop and to do the best they could to support themselves. About not seeing royalties from the film she said that she felt God wanted them to go on living the life they usually led and "attract people to that kind of life . . . and that's that."

Even though she had nothing to do with the play or the film, and was upset that they portrayed the captain as harsh, when he was not (although he did use a whistle!), she said: "It's a good film and it's *almost* completely correct."

Maria didn't stop living after the end of the movie or the death of her husband. She spent over a year touring missions in the South Pacific and had the courage to ask a female cannibal what were the best parts of a human to eat. (The answer is in her book, *Maria*.) She and her family traveled around the world singing, lecturing, and inspiring others. She never lost her faith, passion, or optimism and she died an old, old lady.

Today, you can visit the Trapp Family Lodge in Stowe, Vermont, and still feel Maria's and her family's presence. Her son runs the place. Her daughter and grandchildren lead sing-alongs. Hundreds of thousands of people have gone there to see for themselves if the story was real or not—and to join in the singing in front of the campfire, to go on horse drawn sleigh rides in the winter wonderland of the mountains, to visit the chapel that her son, Werner, built to the blessed Virgin Mary after he survived World War II. The Trapps are making a decent living, but not a decadent one. For those who come here, it's like a pilgrimage to a place where faith and love overcome all obstacles, where the hills *are* alive with the sound of music. And where they find out that the real story is even more dramatic, more romantic, and more extraordinary than the movie.

At the end of the documentary of her life, as she is walking on the streets of Salzburg for the last time, Maria says, "I feel like in a story. A really beautiful story. Which happened to be true."

IN THE END

～◦

Writing this book was a true pleasure. As mother and daughter working together, it was fabulous! And we still enjoy each other's company tremendously. We practiced what we preached and it worked.

To summarize what we have learned during the research and writing of this book:

We can't go back. We can only go forward. While it's tempting to think the past holds some secret answer to all our problems, and that if you just find the original text of some ancient sacred book all the answers will be revealed, the truth is we are all on a journey and we are all evolving. There are some answers in the past, but you'll find more answers now and in the future. The people who created our ideas of God were not perfect, and they were doing the best they could at the time. But ancient values and issues should not hold us back from creating something new and something better.

It's in our hands. We have the power to change the world, our world. We have power in how we raise our children. We have the power to speak up and make changes. And while it's tempting to blame men, the truth is we have been just as responsible. We fought amongst ourselves instead of fighting against the situations. We suffered and sacrificed with "dignity" rather than reaching into our scrappy souls and putting up a fuss. And then, instead of remembering how long and hard it's taken us to get here, we let ourselves forget and take it for granted. It's in our hands.

The true power is in education. There is a reason why women have been prevented for millennia from getting an education. Once our minds are informed, it's hard to hold us back. We are curious. We are smart. We are able to discover and invent new things. But if we are taught to be closed-minded and fearful, we will be. If we are taught to be open-minded and courageous, we will be. If we are taught that war and domination equal power, we will live in a world of conflict. If we are taught that love and harmony equal power, we will live in a world of peace. This is not an issue of choosing between church and state. Religion has no ownership of love and governments have no dominion over our hearts. We believe it's time for a new morality, one that extends beyond any religion and crosses all national, economic, and spiritual lines, one that touches our inner belief in human decency.

There is absolutely no reason to feel guilty about pleasure. All the scientific and medical studies show that pleasure is not the problem, our attitudes about it are. When you dig down deep, it's easy to see how our predisposition to feeling guilty has kept us safely under control. It's time to stop the guilt and start a pleasure revolution in our own lives.

We would also like to thank the amazing women who took the time to talk to us about their lives and our ideas. We were struck by some similarities shared by our pleasure revolutionaries, including those who are no longer living.

All of them have a strong belief and optimism about the potential for human decency and goodness. Whether practicing a religion or "raging atheists," they had a spirit of questioning and openness about their beliefs. Many of them prayed to an unknown life force.

None of them tried to be perfect. In fact, there is a delightful sense of acceptance of their own humanness and imperfection. They were passionate. They were fighters. They were funny. They were struggling and searching. They were absolutely perfect in their imperfection.

Many of them had very hard lives, but they didn't let this stop them from finding pleasure. They never considered themselves victims. In some cases, it's even hard to imagine how difficult their lives must have been —and yet they overcame their circumstances and succeeded tremendously.

Finally, *they all followed their heart and believed in love,* no matter what the obstacles, rules, social systems, men, or any church told them. They took a stand for what they believe in and because of that we are all deeply indebted for their lives and their contribution.

From the bottom of our hearts, we thank the pleasure revolutionaries past and present, known and unknown, public and personal. We promise we won't let you down.

ACKNOWLEDGMENTS

We would like to thank Mark Kintzel, for his amazing ability to keep us organized, scheduled, *and* to deal with crying fits. Thanks to everyone at Rodale, Inc., especially Steve Murphy, for their patience and support while we wrote the book and for helping us get the word out. Thanks to the whole Rodale family, for being there for us and with us, from the very beginning.

We would also like to thank Georgene Bleiler, for being our second mother, our stability, and our consistent caregiver.

Thanks go to Kathy Robbins, for her initial advice, our agent Linda Loewenthal, for her enthusiasm and courage, and our editor, Leslie Meredith, for loving our book and being a great editor. Thanks to the whole team at Free Press for understanding our book, and feeling so strongly about it.

Thanks to all the women we have met and talked to who have shared their stories, their pain, and their pleasure.

Maya would like to thank Alex and her friends for their laughter and love.

Most of all, we would like to thank Lou, for his tolerance, support, and wisdom—even though we're heretics, and even when we don't deserve it.

INDEX